Recent Advances in Trauma and Orthopaedic Surgery

Recent Advances in Trauma and Orthopaedic Surgery

Guest Editors

Konstantinos Tsikopoulos
Panagiotis Givissis

MDPI • Basel • Beijing • Wuhan • Barcelona • Belgrade • Novi Sad • Cluj • Manchester

Guest Editors

Konstantinos Tsikopoulos
1st Department of Pharmacology
Aristotle University of Thessaloniki
Thessaloniki
Greece

Panagiotis Givissis
1st Department of Pharmacology
Aristotle University of Thessaloniki
Thessaloniki
Greece

Editorial Office
MDPI AG
Grosspeteranlage 5
4052 Basel, Switzerland

This is a reprint of the Special Issue, published open access by the journal *Journal of Clinical Medicine* (ISSN 2077-0383), freely accessible at: https://www.mdpi.com/journal/jcm/special_issues/1STP95MLAU.

For citation purposes, cite each article independently as indicated on the article page online and as indicated below:

Lastname, A.A.; Lastname, B.B. Article Title. *Journal Name* **Year**, *Volume Number*, Page Range.

ISBN 978-3-7258-4873-7 (Hbk)
ISBN 978-3-7258-4874-4 (PDF)
https://doi.org/10.3390/books978-3-7258-4874-4

Contents

Journal of
Clinical Medicine

MDPI

Systematic Review

Percutaneous Fixation for Traumatic Symphysis Pubis Disruption—Are the Results Superior Compared to Open Techniques? A Systematic Review and Meta-Analysis of Clinical and Biomechanical Outcomes

Dimitrios Kitridis [1,*], Konstantinos Tsikopoulos [2], Panagiotis Givissis [1] and Byron Chalidis [1]

1 1st Orthopaedic Department, School of Medicine, Faculty of Health Science, Aristotle University of Thessaloniki, 54124 Thessaloniki, Greece; pgivissis@gmail.com (P.G.); byronchalidis@gmail.com (B.C.)
2 1st Department of Pharmacology, School of Medicine, Faculty of Health Science, Aristotle University of Thessaloniki, 54124 Thessaloniki, Greece; kostastsikop@gmail.com
* Correspondence: dkitridis@gmail.com

Abstract: Introduction: Open reduction and reconstruction plate and screws fixation (RPSF) is considered the gold standard for the treatment of traumatic symphysis pubis diastasis (SPD). Percutaneous cannulated screw fixation (PCSF) has recently gained popularity as it may reduce operative time and morbidity. The current systematic review aims to compare the clinical and radiological outcomes of PCSF and RPSF in traumatic SPD and analyze the biomechanical effectiveness of PCSF. Material and Methods: The Medline, Scopus, and Cochrane databases were searched until February 2023. The primary outcomes were the incidence of implant failure and revision surgery and the amount of displacement of symphysis pubis. Secondary outcomes were the intraoperative blood loss, the scar length, the operative time, the wound infection, and the patients' functional improvement. Results: Six clinical trial studies with a total of 184 patients and nine biomechanical studies were included. There was no significant difference between the two groups regarding the incidence of implant failure, the prevalence of revision surgery, and the amount of postoperative loss of reduction ($p > 0.05$ for all outcomes). The intraoperative blood loss (14.9 ± 4.2 mL for PCSF versus 162.7 ± 47.6 mL for PCSF, $p < 0.001$) and the incision length (1.7 ± 0.9 mL for PCSF versus 8 ± 1.4 mL for PCSF, $p < 0.001$) were significantly lower after PCSF. The mean operative time was 37 ± 19.1 min for PCSF and 68.9 ± 13.6 min for RPSF ($p < 0.001$). The infection rate was less frequent in the PCSF group (3% for PCSF versus 14.3% for RPSF, $p = 0.01$). One clinical trial reported better functional recovery after PCSF. In all biomechanical studies, the threshold for implant failure was beyond the applied forces corresponding to daily activities. Conclusions: PCSF for traumatic SPD is associated with less operative time, less blood loss, and a lower infection rate when compared to conventional plate techniques without increasing the incidence of postoperative fixation failure and revision surgery. Moreover, PCSF has been proven to be biomechanically sufficient for stabilization. Therefore, it should be considered an efficient and viable alternative for the reconstruction of SPD when closed reduction can be adequately achieved.

Keywords: traumatic; pubic symphysis diastasis; pelvic fractures; percutaneous cannulated screw; minimally invasive; reconstruction plate; biomechanics

1. Introduction

The incidence rate of pelvic and acetabular fractures is increasing as a result of the increased occurrence of high-energy injuries caused by traffic accidents or falling from high places [1,2]. The mortality risk following pelvic fractures ranges from 5% to 20%, which is a remaining challenge in the field of orthopedic and trauma surgery [2]. The modified Tile classification has been widely used to describe the fracture patterns, allowing assessment of the stability of the pelvic ring [1]. Symphysis pubis diastasis (SPD) occurs in approximately 24% of pelvic fractures and may be associated with other pelvic ring injuries [1,2]. Simple SPD, named the "open book" lesion, is rotationally unstable and is characterized as type B1 according to the Tile classification [2]. Widening of the symphysis pubis (SP) greater than 25 mm implicates that the anterior sacroiliac ligaments are mostly damaged and is considered an indication for surgery [3], which may be performed either alone or simultaneously with posterior pelvic ring fixation according to the integrity of the posterior pelvis [4,5].

Open reduction and reconstruction plate and screws fixation (RPSF) via a Pfannenstiel approach is considered till now the standard treatment for unstable SP injury, providing relatively easy access to the anterior pelvic ring and a low incidence of incisional hernia [6]. However, the technique has several disadvantages. Although the anatomy of the anterior pelvis is well-described, the exposure of the symphysis pubis may cause significant blood loss, as well as neural and vascular injuries [7]. The lateral extension of the incision can damage the inguinal canal contents and lead to chronic pain disability [8]. Furthermore, wound problems, especially in obese and diabetic patients, and heterotopic bone formation may be encountered [9].

With the improvement of intraoperative imaging, several alternative less traumatic fixation methods have been recently introduced and gained popularity as they could reduce operative time and morbidity. Minimally invasive [10] or endoscopic plate fixation [11,12], percutaneous cannulated screw fixation (PCSF) [8,13], Endobutton technique for dynamic fixation [10], and tape suture fixation [14] promise not only adequate stability of the disrupted anterior pelvic ring but also smaller skin incisions, less soft tissue trauma, and minimal blood loss [2]. However, published reports of PCSF for SPD are quite rare, and the overall value and superiority of the technique remain unclear. The purpose of the current systematic review is to compare the outcomes and complication rates of PCSF and RPSF in traumatic SPD and present the available evidence regarding the biomechanical effectiveness and safety of different PCSF options.

2. Material and Methods

2.1. Search Strategy and Eligibility Criteria

The present review was performed in agreement with the Preferred Reporting Items for Systematic Reviews and Meta-Analyses (PRISMA) guidelines, albeit not a priori registered [15]. A systematic search of the Pubmed, Scopus, and Cochrane Central Register of Controlled Trials databases was performed until February 2023. The following search string was used: "(pubi*) AND (symphys*) AND (percutaneous OR minimally)". No date limits or additional filters were utilized. The references of the included articles were further manually searched for additional studies. Two authors independently screened the relevant records for inclusion.

Articles were included if they met one of the following criteria:

1. The study reported clinical outcomes after the application of PCSF either alone or in comparison with RPSF for traumatic SPD in patients 16 years of age or older.
2. The study reported biomechanical or anatomical properties of PCSF in cadaveric or software simulation studies.

Articles were excluded if they met the following criteria:

1. The report was a conference abstract.
2. The study did not present clinical or biomechanical data, such as reviews and letters to the editor.
3. The study evaluated nontraumatic SPD.
4. The study was not written in the English language.

2.2. Data Extraction

Two authors independently reviewed and extracted data from the selected articles including studies' (type of study, year, country) and patients' characteristics, surgical interventions, outcomes, complications, and length of follow-up period. The primary outcomes of the study were the incidence of implant failure and revision surgery, as well as the amount of post-surgery displacement of the symphysis pubis as measured at the immediate postoperative and latest follow-up radiographs. Secondary outcomes were the intraoperative blood loss, the scar length, the operative time, the incidence of wound infection, and the patients' functional outcomes. Information considering the biomechanical efficacy of the fixation techniques was based on the threshold values for implant failure and specifically whether the fixated symphysis could withstand the applied forces corresponding to daily activities of sitting, standing, and walking. Furthermore, data from anatomical studies were analyzed also regarding the distance of the screws' trajectories from major structures and whether any injuries were reported.

2.3. Quality Assessment

For clinical case series studies, the Moga et al. [16] checklist was used (a score of 13–18 indicates high quality, 7–12 moderate, and 0–6 low quality). The Coleman et al. [17] score was applied for the quality assessment of clinical comparative studies (a scale of 0 to 100; a score of 100% is considered the perfect score and indicates high quality).

Regarding the biomechanical and anatomical studies, there is currently no validated quality appraisal tool. The assessment was based on a modified checklist developed by Dewan et al. [18]. This checklist is a combination of the relevant elements of the Critical Appraisal Skills Programme (CASP) tool and the Quality Appraisal for Cadaveric Studies (QUACS) scale [19,20].

2.4. Statistical Analysis

The meta-analysis was performed with the Review Manager software (RevMan Version 5.3, Copenhagen: The Nordic Cochrane Centre, The Cochrane Collaboration, 2014) using the effect size of standardized mean difference according to the inverse variance method and a random-effects model because of the anticipated heterogeneity across studies [21]. Only studies with direct comparisons were included in the meta-analysis. If a meta-analysis was not feasible, continuous data were pooled using weights according to each study's sample size and compared using the two-tailed Student's *t*-test assuming equal variances between the two groups. Categorical outcomes were compared using the chi-squared test. Microsoft Excel version 16 and IBM Statistical Package for Social Sciences (SPSS) software version 24 were used for the analyses. The level of significance was set at $p < 0.05$.

3. Results

The initial database and manual search identified 547 articles, of which 223 were duplicates and 275 were excluded using the titles and abstracts. Finally, 15 articles including six clinical and nine biomechanical studies fulfilled the eligibility criteria and were considered to be relevant for this review. The flow chart of the selection process is presented in Figure 1.

3.1. Characteristics of Clinical Studies

Six clinical studies described PCSF for traumatic SPD [2,3,7,22–24]. In more detail, one prospective randomized trial [22] and one retrospective non-randomized trial [2] compared PCSF with RPSF, one prospective randomized comparative trial compared PCSF with a TightRope (Arthrex, Naples, FL, USA) device combined with an external fixator [7], one retrospective case series study evaluated PCSF [23], and two retrospective case series studies evaluated computer-navigated PCSF [3,24]. These studies enrolled 219 patients in total, and the number of patients completing the follow-up assessments was 114 for PCSF and 70 for RPSF. The publication dates ranged between 2009 and 2022. Five studies were conducted in Asia [2,3,7,22,24], and one in the United States of America [23]. The clinical studies' characteristics are presented in Table 1.

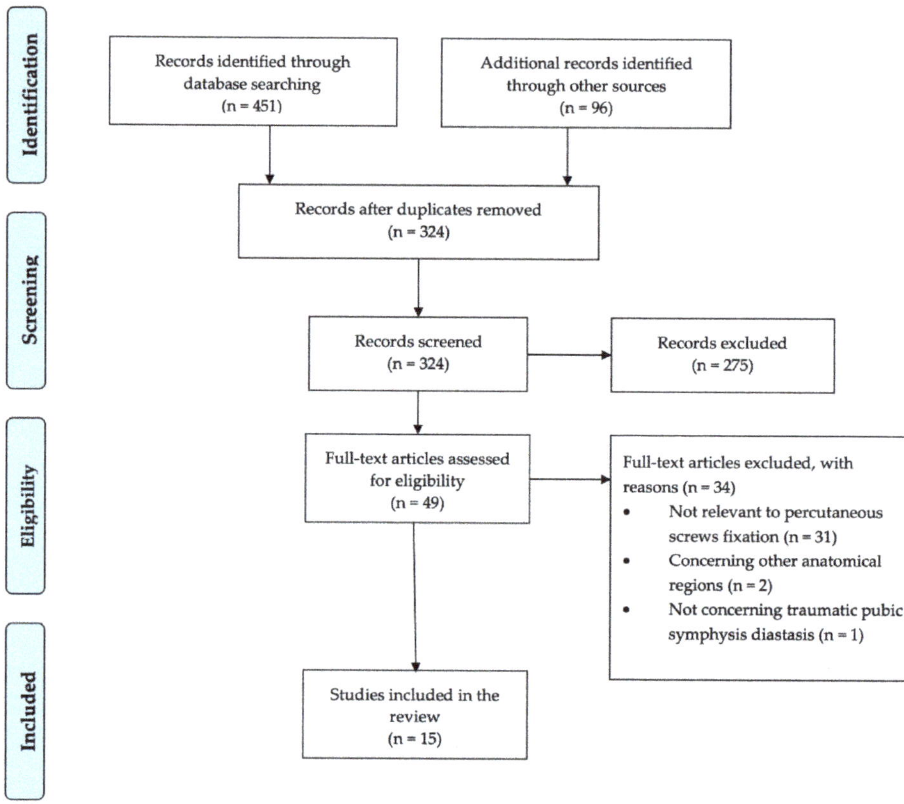

Figure 1. PRISMA flow diagram of the study.

Table 1. Characteristics of the included clinical studies.

Study	Technique	N	Mean Age (yr)	Males/Females	Mean Follow-Up (mo)
Chan et al. [24], 2022	Single or dual 6.5 mm PCSF	13	57.9 (24–95)	8/7	At least 6
Chen et al. [22], 2012	A. Single 7.3 mm PCSF	41	32 ± 9	29/12	21 (18–26)
	B. RPSF	43	26 ± 11	33/9	
Eakin et al. [23], 2022	Single or dual 5.5, 6.5, or 7.3 mm PCSF	12	44 (16–76)	10/2	15 (10.7–27.7)
Feng et al. [7], 2016	A. Single 6.5 mm PCSF	16	33.2 ± 5.8	11/5	15 (12–20)
	B. Tightrope and ex-fix	10	32.5 ± 6.2	7/3	
Mu et al. [3], 2016	Single or dual crossed 7.3 mm PCSF, computer navigation	8	40.9 ± 17.9	6/2	16.1 ± 2.5
Yu et al. [2], 2015	A. Single 6.5 mm PCSF	24	33.4 ± 9.1	15/9	29.4 ± 8.8
	B. RPSF	27	34.8 ± 11.7	19/8	

PCSF: percutaneous cannulated screw fixation; RPSF: reconstruction plate and screws fixation.

3.2. Percutaneous Fixation Technique

Regarding PCSF, closed reduction of the SPD was achieved by using two Schanz pins that were inserted into both iliac crests and large pointed reduction clamps [2,3,7,22]. Afterward, a K-wire was introduced between the pubic tubercle and the ipsilateral superior ramus and was forwarded to the contralateral superior ramus under fluoroscopy guidance. Then, a 6.5 or 7.3 mm short-threaded cannulated screw was inserted along the K-wire [2,3,7,22,23]. In the case of concomitant posterior pelvic disruption, posterior fixation was also performed with percutaneous sacroiliac screws. Mu et al. [3] and Chan et al. [24] used computer navigation and implanted a second screw to achieve improved stability if anatomy and execution were possible. In more detail, in cases of posterior pelvic disruption or multiple rami fractures, Mu et al. [3] inserted a second crossed screw from the base of the pubic tubercle to the superior part of the opposite side body of the pubis. Furthermore, Chen et al. [22] applied the PCSF technique in patients with vertical shear pelvic injuries, after correcting the vertical displacement with 10–12 kg supracondylar traction for several days.

3.3. Characteristics of Biomechanical and Anatomical Studies

Nine studies published from 2012 to 2022 investigated the biomechanical properties of PCSF [2,25–32]. Four studies utilized cadaveric specimens [25–28], two conducted finite elements analyses [2,29], two performed both cadaveric and finite element analyses [30,31], and one utilized composite pelvis models [32]. Five trials were conducted in Asia [2,27,29–31], two in Europe [25,26], and one in the United States of America [32]; one included authors from both Asia and the United States of America [28] (Table 2).

Table 2. Characteristics of the included biomechanical and anatomical studies.

Study	Fracture Simulation	Implants	Testing Method	Outcomes	Specimens	Results/Conclusions
Cano-Luis et al. [25], 2012	Tile B1	Dual 6.5 mm PCSF	Axial load 300N (dual-leg standing)	Displacement of pubic symphysis	10 cadavers	PCSF biomechanically sufficient
Gonzálvez et al. [26], 2016	Tile B1	A. Dual 6.5 mm PCSF B. 3.5 mm superior RPSF	Axial load 300N (dual-leg standing)	Displacement of pubic symphysis	9 cadavers	PCSF more stable than RPSF
Liu et al. [31], 2022	Intact pelvis	Single 7.5 mm PCSF	Determination of the optimal insertion point and safe channels of screws	Screws diameter and length, distance between screw and anterior inferior iliac spine, coronal, sagittal, and horizontal plane angles	A. 3D finite element model analysis B. 16 cadavers	Screw length 47.0 ± 2.0 mm (M) and 39.8 ± 3.9 mm (F), diameter 7.1 ± 0.4 mm (M) and 6.1 ± 0.4 mm (F), distance between screw and AIIS 5.5 ± 0.5 mm (M) and 5.6 ± 0.7 mm (F), angle of coronal plane 55.9° ± 1.3° (M) and 50.7° ± 1.5° (F), angle of sagittal plane 26.7° ± 0.5° (M) and 24.1° ± 0.9° (F), and angle of horizontal plane 64.8° ± 0.6° (M) and 58.8° ± 0.8° (F). Safe screw insertion 5 mm above AIIS, and 10 mm outside the midline of the symphysis pubis.

Table 2. *Cont.*

Study	Fracture Simulation	Implants	Testing Method	Outcomes	Specimens	Results/Conclusions
O'Neill et al. [32], 2022	Tile C1	A. 6.5 mm 4-hole plate and 6.5 mm S1 transsacral screw B. Single 6.5 mm cannulated stain-less steel screw and 6.5 mm S1 transsacral screw	7 mm vertical compressive displacement through the sacrum at a rate of 2 mm/s (single-leg standing)	Displacement and rotation in 3 dimensions at the sacroiliac joint and pubic symphysis, stiffness at maximum stroke distance	A. 4 B. 4	There was no significant difference in net displacement at both sacroiliac joint and pubic symphysis. There was significantly less rotation but more dis-placement in the screw group in the Z-axis. The screw group showed increased stiffness compared with the plate group.
Sun et al. [27], 2016	Intact pelvis	Dual crossed 6.5 mm PCSF	Optimization of the secure trajectory of crossed screws using computer navigation	Trajectory, mean screw length, distance from surrounding major structures	15 cadavers	Mean screw length 7.0 ± 4.2 and 7.1 ± 3.8 cm. Minimum distance between entry point and spermatic cord (fallopian arch in the female) was 9 mm. All screw corridors were intact. Computer navigation is reliable for PCSF. The trajectories of crossed screws are reliable and safe.
Xu et al. [28], 2016	Intact pelvis	A. Single 7.3 mm PCSF/fluoroscopy B. Single 7.3 mm PCSF/2D fluoro-scopic navigation C. Single 7.3 mm PCSF/3D fluoro-scopic navigation	Determination of the accuracy of screw position, instrumentation time, and fluoroscopic time	Malposition rate, mean instrumentation time, mean fluoroscopic time	6 cadavers	3D fluoroscopic navigation showed a higher accuracy rate in positioning and a shorter instrumentation time. The fluoroscopic time was the shortest in 2D fluoroscopic navigation.
Yao et al. [29], 2015	Tile B1	A. Superior RPSF B. Superior and ante-rior RPSF C. Single 7.3 mm PCSF D. Dual crossed PCSF (7.3 and 6.5 mm) E. Dual par-allel PCSF (7.3 and 6.5 mm)	A. Axial load 500 N (dual-leg standing) B. Axial load 750 N (single-leg standing) C. Axial load 500 N, torque 7 Nm (rotation)	Construct stiffness, incremental micromotion of anterior and posterior pelvic ring, incremental rotational angle of anterior pelvic ring	3D finite element model analysis	Dual crossed PCSF and dual RPSF more stable methods

Table 2. *Cont.*

Study	Fracture Simulation	Implants	Testing Method	Outcomes	Specimens	Results/Conclusions
Yu et al. [2], 2015	Tile B1	A. Single 6.5 mm PCSF B. 3.5 mm superior RPSF	Axial load 600 N (single-leg standing)	Whole stress, displacement of the bilateral pelvis, stress analysis of implants	3D finite element model analysis	Both PCSF and RPSF biomechanically adequate
Yu et al. [30], 2015	Intact pelvis	Single 6.5 mm PCSF	Optimization of the secure trajectory of screws	Distance from surrounding major structures, screw trajectory parameters	A. 13 cadavers B. 3D finite element model analysis	Distance between round ligament of the uterus and pubic tubercle was 4.408 ± 0.304 mm, and between spermatic cord and pubic tubercle was 5.196 ± 0.251 mm. Study on parameters of screw channel in PCSF can improve the accuracy of the screw placement.

PCSF: percutaneous cannulated screw fixation; RPSF: reconstruction plate and screws fixation; M: males; F: females; AIIS: anterior inferior iliac spine.

3.4. Quality Assessment

Two clinical studies provided level II evidence [7,22], one provided level III evidence [2], and three provided level IV evidence [3,23,24]. The comparative clinical trials were rated with a mean Coleman methodology score of 82.3% (range 63–93%) [2,7,22]. The case series studies by Eakin et al. [23] and Chan et al. [24] were of high quality (14 out of 18 points), and the study by Mu et al. [3] was of moderate quality (10 out of 18 points) according to the Moga score.

All biomechanical and anatomical studies utilized mechanical setup and parameters, which were representative of the in vivo biological conditions (Table 2). However, most studies did not explore repetitive loadings or tissue adaptation over time. The detailed critical appraisal of the biomechanical studies according to the checklist developed by Dewan et al. [18] is presented in Table 3.

3.5. Primary Outcomes

Implant failure was reported in 11 patients (9.6%) after PCSF and in 10 patients (14.3%) after RPSF. However, this difference did not reach statistical significance (p = 0.34). The incidence of revision surgery due to postoperative displacement and construct failure was similar in both groups as it was required in four patients in the PCSF group (3.5%) and in seven patients in the RPSF group (10%), (p = 0.07) (Table 4).

Table 3. Quality assessment of the included biomechanical and anatomical studies.

Study	Objective Stated	Appropriate Study Design	Basic Information about Specimens	Conditions of Specimens	Study Protocol Clearly Stated	Exposure Accurately Measured	Outcome Accurately Measured	Results Presented Thoroughly	Stats Appropriate	Limitations Discussed	Clinical Implications Discussed	Conclusions in Keeping with Results	Results Fit with Other Studies
Cano-Luis et al. [25], 2012	✓	✓	✓	✓	✓	✓	✓	✓	✓	✓	✓	✓	✓
Gonzálvez et al. [26], 2016	✓	✓	✓	✓	✓	✓	✓	✓	✓	✓	✓	✓	✓
Liu et al. [31], 2022	✓	✓	✓	✓	✓	✓	✓	✓	✓	✓	✓	✓	✓
O'Neill et al. [32], 2022	✓	✓	✓	✓	✓	✓	✓	✓	✓	✓	✓	✓	✓
Sun et al. [27], 2016	✓	✓	✓	✓	✓	✓	✓	✓	✓	✓	✓	✓	✓
Xu et al. [28], 2016	✓	✓	✗	✗	✓	✓	✓	✓	✓	✗	✓	✓	✓
Yao et al. [29], 2015	✓	✓	N/A	N/A	✓	✓	✓	✓	✗	✓	✓	✓	✓
Yu et al. [2], 2015 (1)	✓	✓	N/A	N/A	✓	✓	✓	✓	✗*	✓	✓	✓	✓
Yu et al. [30], 2015 (2)	✓	✓	✓	✓	✓	✓	✓	✓	✗	✓	✓	✓	✓

N/A: Not applicable; *: Only for finite elements analysis.

Table 4. Complications reported in the included clinical studies.

Study	Technique	N	Implant Failure	Revision Surgery	Wound Infection
Chan et al. [24], 2022	PCSF	13	-	-	-
Chen et al. [22], 2012	A. PCSF	41	5	2	2
	B. RPSF	43	8	6	8
Eakin et al. [23], 2022	PCSF	12	-	-	-
Feng et al. [7], 2016	A. PCSF	16	3	1	-
	B. Tightrope and ex-fix	10	1	-	1
Mu et al. [3], 2016	PCSF	8	-	-	-
Yu et al. [2], 2015	A. PCSF	24	2	1	1
	B. RPSF	27	2	1	2

PCSF: percutaneous cannulated screw fixation; RPSF: reconstruction plate and screws fixation; N/R: not reported.

The mean difference between immediate postoperative and final follow-up SP width was 0.62 ± 1.33 mm and 1.17 ± 2.45 mm after PCSF and RPSF, respectively. However, this change was not statistically significant (p = 0.07).

3.6. Secondary Outcomes

The mean intraoperative blood loss for PCSF was 14.9 ± 4.2 mL, while for RPSF it was 162.7 ± 47.6 mL. The mean skin incision length was 1.7 ± 0.9 cm for PCSF and 8 ± 1.4 cm for RPSF. The meta-analysis demonstrated a statistically significant difference in favor of PCSF for both parameters ($p < 0.001$ for both outcomes, Figure 2).

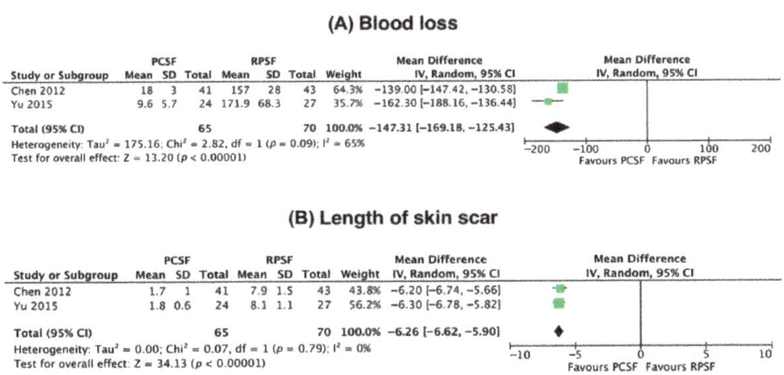

Figure 2. Forest plots demonstrating the mean difference of intraoperative blood loss (**A**) and length of skin scar (**B**) between percutaneous cannulated screw fixation (PCSF) reconstruction plate and screws fixation (RPSF). Chen et al. [15], 2012; Yu et al. [2], 2015.

The mean operative time was significantly shorter for PCSF than for RPSF (37 ± 19.1 versus 68.9 ± 13.6 min, respectively, $p < 0.001$). However, the duration of surgery was significantly increased after the application of computer navigation for PCSF (57 ± 12.5 minutes, $p < 0.01$, when compared to non-navigated PCSF).

Superficial infection was more frequent after RPSF rather than PCSF (10 patients, 14.3%, versus three patients, 3%, respectively, Table 4) ($p < 0.01$). All patients were treated conservatively with antibiotics and frequent wound dressing changes. No case of deep infection was reported.

Regarding functional outcomes, four studies reported a scoring system described by Majeed et al. [33], which utilized clinical information such as pain, sitting, sexual intercourse, walking, and working [2,7,22,24]. Two studies compared PCSF with RPSF [2,22], and one study compared PCSF with a TightRope technique [7]. Only the study by Chen et al. [22], which compared PCSF with RPSF, reported better functional recovery after PCSF (Table 5).

Table 5. Functional outcomes according to Majeed scoring system.

Study	Technique	N	Excellent (>85)	Good (70–84)	Fair (55–69)	Poor (<55)	p
Chan et al. [24], 2022	PCSF	12	2	2	4	4	-
Chen et al. [22], 2012	PCSF	41	23	12	5	1	0.01
	RPSF	43	10	24	5	3	
Feng et al. [7], 2016	PCSF	16	11	4	1	-	n.s.
	Tightrope and ex-fix	10	7	3	-	-	
Yu et al. [2], 2015	PCSF	24	18	5	1	-	n.s.
	RPSF	27	18	7	2	-	

PCSF: percutaneous cannulated screw fixation; RPSF: reconstruction plate and screws fixation; n.s.: non-significant.

3.7. Biomechanical Outcomes

The research setups utilized axial loads imitating single- and dual-leg standing [2,25,26,32], as well as axial loads combined with rotational torque loads [29]. In all biomechanical studies, the threshold of failure was beyond the applied forces of daily activities and standing. In the comparative biomechanical studies, the cannulated screws provided comparable biomechanical properties to plate fixation [2,26,29,32]. Overall, the authors concluded that PCSF was biomechanically adequate to resist failure after surgery (Table 2).

Four anatomical studies assessed the accuracy and safety of screw positioning by determining the trajectories of the screws and the relevant distances from the surrounding major anatomical structures [27,28,30,31]. The studies did not report any inadvertent injury of neurovascular or soft tissue elements and consequently verified that fluoroscopy guidance may guarantee the accurate introduction of the screws.

4. Discussion

The present systematic review showed that PCSF is a successful alternative for the treatment of traumatic SPD. According to the available data, there is no significant difference between standard open and percutaneous fixation techniques regarding the incidence of implant failure, the prevalence of revision surgery, and postoperative SP displacement. Compared to RPSF, PCSF has been associated with shorter operative time, less intraoperative blood loss, and shorter skin incision length ($p < 0.001$ for all parameters). However, the functional outcomes and the infection rates were found not to differ significantly across the study groups.

Based on the available clinical studies, we noticed a low rate of implant failure after PCSF, which was similar to the traditional plate fixation method (10% and 14.3%, respectively, $p = 0.38$). Eakin et al. [23] reported only one case of loss of reduction after 10 weeks postoperatively among the 12 patients treated with PCSF due to SPD. Interestingly, there was no radiographic evidence of screw breakage. Both Chen et al. [22] and Yu et al. [2] found similar rates of implant failure between the PCSF and RPSF groups ($p = 0.39$ and 1, respectively). Moreover, Chen et al. [22] recommended earlier hardware removal following PCSF since they considered that screw fixation was biomechanically more stable than RPSF. They advocated screw removal after 10 months postoperatively, particularly in young female patients to facilitate uneventful childbirth.

According to the current systematic review, the mean operative time is shorter in PCSF when compared to open fixation techniques ($p < 0.001$). On the other hand, some minimally invasive techniques are quite demanding, and therefore the surgical time may be prolonged. Specifically, Feng et al. [7] reported that the Tightrope technique combined with external fixation lasted 48.5 ± 9.4 min. Similarly, Mu et al. [3] recorded a longer operative time in eight patients with SPD who were operated on with a percutaneous lag screw under a fluoroscopy-based Iso-C3D computerized navigation system (57 ± 12.5 min). However, due to the paucity of available data, more studies are necessary to establish the beneficial effect of computer navigation in PCSF.

Among the proposed benefits of a minimally invasive procedure are reduced blood loss and operative time. Chen et al. [22] reported that patients treated with PCSF exhibited less intraoperative blood loss (18 ± 3 mL for PCSF versus 157 ± 28 mL for RPSF, $p < 0.01$) and extensive exposure (mean skin incision length for PCSF 1.7 ± 1 cm versus 7.9 ± 1.5 cm for RPSF, $p < 0.001$) than those who received plate fixation. Similarly, Yu et al. [2] enrolled patients with isolated Tile type B1 injuries and showed that the blood loss and the length of the skin incision in the PCSF group were significantly smaller than those in the RPSF group (blood loss 9.6 ± 5.7 mL versus 171.9 ± 68.3 mL, skin incision length for PCSF 1.8 ± 0.6 cm versus 8.1 ± 1.1 cm, respectively, $p < 0.001$ for both outcomes). Regarding the parameter of functional improvement, only Chen et al. [22] reported better and quicker functional recovery in favor of PCSF. This can be explained by the limited tissue trauma and subsequent faster healing process. The iatrogenic injury caused by detachment of the distal insertion of the rectus abdominis muscle to obtain adequate exposure of the SP during RPSF may delay patients' recovery and predispose to abdominal hernia formation [34].

In terms of fixation stability and potential postoperative displacement, the comparable results between the two techniques reflect the effectiveness of the PCSF, which has been also documented in biomechanical studies. Recent literature has shown that the forces across the disrupted symphysis pubis are transmitted through the plate during the rehabilitation phase [35]. The plate–screw construct represents an eccentric–extramedullary fixation of the SP, in contrast with the cannulated screws only. The latter option acts as an intramedullary device and carries the biomechanical benefit of decreasing the number of stresses transmitted by the implant. Therefore, the cannulated screws may result in a lower failure rate [36]. Cano-Luis et al. [25] compared the biomechanical properties of the intact symphysis pubis and SPD fixed with PCSF and found that there was no significant difference in the mean displacement after the application of an axial load of 300N ($p > 0.7$). The authors advocated that the cannulated screws could effectively resist rotational forces and offer adequate stability of the anterior pelvic ring. Gonzálvez et al. [26] performed a biomechanical study in fresh human pelvis specimens simulating an AO B1.1 injury that was fixed with two cannulated screws or a 6-hole non-locked plate. After axial load application of 300N, the cannulated screws fixation was associated with better stability and superior biomechanical behavior compared to plate fixation.

Dual fixation has been also recommended to improve the strength of the construct and minimize the incidence of loss of reduction. Yao et al. [29], in a 3-dimensional finite element model of SPD (Tile type B1), observed that dual fixation of SPD with a superior and anterior plate (dual-plate) or crossed dual cannulated screws (cross-screw) offered better anterior and posterior pelvic stability than single superior plate or single cannulated screw constructs. However, the clinical implications of their study are yet to be determined. Yu et al. [2], in another finite element analysis study, found that PCSF and RPSF were equally adequate and effective for SP fixation as the maximum observed displacement of SP was 0.643 and 0.408 mm, respectively.

When considering the safety of the PCSF technique, the published studies did not report any injury to the major structures and consequently verified that fluoroscopy guidance may guarantee the accurate introduction of the screws. Sun et al. [27] in a cadaveric study measured the distance of the screw corridors from the nearby major structures. They reported a minimum distance between the entry point and the spermatic cord (fallopian arch in the female) of 9 mm. Similarly, Yu et al. [30] found that the mean distance between the pubic tubercle and the round ligament of the uterus or the spermatic cord was 4.408 ± 0.304 mm, and 5.196 ± 0.251 mm, respectively. On the subject of the appropriate screw entry points, Liu et al. [31] provided the anatomical basis for implant insertion using a finite elements model as well as 16 cadaveric specimens. They observed that regardless of patients' gender, the introduction of the screws at approximately 5 mm above the anterior inferior iliac spine and 10 mm outside the midline of the symphysis pubis was a safe procedure.

Although PCSF is applied mostly in Tile type B1 injuries, its indications may be further expanded to SPD injuries combined with vertical instability of the sacroiliac joint [3,22]. Chen et al. [22] corrected the vertical pelvis displacement by application of 10–12 kg supracondylar traction for several days before surgery. Moreover, in the presence of SPD along with pubic rami fractures, another percutaneously inserted screw towards the broken ramus may be necessary to stabilize the anterior ring. [3,22]. However, percutaneous fixation should be applied with caution or even avoided in case of regional infection, bladder injury, or incarceration during closed SPD reduction and open or comminuted fractures [3,22]. Obesity is also considered a relative contraindication for PCSF, as screw insertion may be hindered by the circumference of the thighs [3]. A figure-of-four position of the contralateral lower limb with the manual pressure of the contralateral proximal thigh are proposed to minimize the amount of soft tissue blocking the trajectory and to increase the amount of working space for the surgeon [24].

Limitations

The current study has some limitations. From a methodology point of view, all the published data were not comparative, so it was not feasible to perform a meta-analysis with direct comparisons of all outcomes. Moreover, three clinical studies were retrospective and therefore might introduce selection or recall bias. From biomechanical point of view, all the relevant studies simulated a Tile B1 pelvic injury. However, in clinical practice, most of the patients have a combination of SPD with other anterior and/or posterior pelvic injuries. In addition, in a highly urgent and demanding emergency situation, the application of a percutaneous minimal invasive technique might be not as good as it may be in cadaveric studies or controlled operative settings. This can influence the outcomes and the effectiveness of PCSF.

5. Conclusions

PCSF for traumatic SPD has all the advantages of a minimally invasive procedure, including less blood loss, minimal morbidity, and rapid recovery. The technique has been proven biomechanically effective to offer stability to the anterior pelvic ring and should be considered a reliable alternative to conventional plate fixation. Nevertheless, it is a challenging and demanding procedure with a long learning curve and higher intra-operative radiation exposure, and its application should be utilized in specific injury patterns.

Author Contributions: Conceptualization, D.K. and B.C.; methodology, D.K and K.T.; software, D.K.; validation, D.K., K.T. and B.C.; formal analysis, D.K.; writing—original draft preparation, D.K.; writing—review and editing, P.G. and B.C.; visualization, D.K.; supervision, P.G. and B.C.; project administration, B.C. All authors have read and agreed to the published version of the manuscript.

Funding: This research received no external funding.

Institutional Review Board Statement: Not applicable.

Informed Consent Statement: Not applicable.

Data Availability Statement: Not applicable.

Conflicts of Interest: The authors declare no conflict of interest.

References

1. Pohlemann, T.; Bosch, U.; Gänsslen, A.; Tscherne, H. The Hannover Experience in Management of Pelvic Fractures. *Clin. Orthop. Relat. Res.* **1994**, *305*, 69–80. [CrossRef]
2. Yu, K.-H.; Hong, J.-J.; Guo, X.-S.; Zhou, D.-S. Comparison of Reconstruction Plate Screw Fixation and Percutaneous Cannulated Screw Fixation in Treatment of Tile B1 Type Pubic Symphysis Diastasis: A Finite Element Analysis and 10-Year Clinical Experience. *J. Orthop. Surg. Res.* **2015**, *10*, 151. [CrossRef] [PubMed]

3. Mu, W.; Wang, H.; Zhou, D.; Yu, L.; Jia, T.; Li, L. Computer Navigated Percutaneous Screw Fixation for Traumatic Pubic Symphysis Diastasis of Unstable Pelvic Ring Injuries. *Chin. Med. J.* **2009**, *122*, 1699–1703. [PubMed]
4. Phieffer, L.S.; Lundberg, W.P.; Templeman, D.C. Instability of the Posterior Pelvic Ring Associated with Disruption of the Pubic Symphysis. *Orthop. Clin. N. Am.* **2004**, *35*, 445–449. [CrossRef] [PubMed]
5. Putnis, S.E.; Pearce, R.; Wali, U.J.; Bircher, M.D.; Rickman, M.S. Open Reduction and Internal Fixation of a Traumatic Diastasis of the Pubic Symphysis: One-Year Radiological and Functional Outcomes. *J. Bone Joint Surg. Br.* **2011**, *93*, 78–84. [CrossRef]
6. Cole, J.D.; Bolhofner, B.R. Acetabular Fracture Fixation via a Modified Stoppa Limited Intrapelvic Approach. Description of Operative Technique and Preliminary Treatment Results. *Clin. Orthop. Relat. Res.* **1994**, *305*, 112–123. [CrossRef]
7. Feng, Y.; Hong, J.; Guo, X.; Lin, C.; Ling, W.; Zhang, L.; Wang, G. Percutaneous Fixation of Traumatic Pubic Symphysis Diastasis Using a TightRope and External Fixator versus Using a Cannulated Screw. *J. Orthop. Surg. Res.* **2016**, *11*, 62. [CrossRef]
8. Grewal, I.S.; Starr, A.J. What's New in Percutaneous Pelvis Fracture Surgery? *Orthop. Clin. N. Am.* **2020**, *51*, 317–324. [CrossRef]
9. Purcell, K.F.; Bergin, P.F.; Spitler, C.A.; Graves, M.L.; Russell, G.V. Management of Pelvic and Acetabular Fractures in the Obese Patient. *Orthop. Clin. N. Am.* **2018**, *49*, 317–324. [CrossRef]
10. Liu, Z.; Wang, K.; Zhang, K.; Zhou, J.; Zhang, Y. Minimally Invasive Surgery (MIS) of Anterior Ring Fracture Combined with Pubic Symphysis Separation. *Med. Sci. Monit.* **2014**, *20*, 1913–1917. [CrossRef]
11. Kabir, K.; Lingohr, P.; Jaenisch, M.; Hackenberg, R.K.; Sommer, N.; Ossendorff, R.; Welle, K.; Gathen, M. Total Endoscopic Anterior Pelvic Approach (TAPA)-A New Approach to the Internal Fixation of the Symphysis. *Injury* **2022**, *53*, 802–808. [CrossRef]
12. Hartel, M.J.; Althoff, G.; Wolter, S.; Ondruschka, B.; Dietz, E.; Frosch, K.-H.K.; Thiesen, D.M. Full Endoscopic Anterior Intrapelvic Plate Osteosynthesis: A Cadaveric Feasibility Study. *Arch. Orthop. Trauma Surg.* **2022**, *143*, 365–371. [CrossRef]
13. Pierce, T.P.; Issa, K.; Callaghan, J.J.; Wright, C. Traumatic Diastasis of the Pubic Symphysis-A Review of Fixation Method Outcomes. *Surg. Technol. Int.* **2016**, *29*, 265–269.
14. Cavalcanti Kußmaul, A.; Schwaabe, F.; Kistler, M.; Gennen, C.; Andreß, S.; Becker, C.A.; Böcker, W.; Greiner, A. Novel Minimally Invasive Tape Suture Osteosynthesis for Instabilities of the Pubic Symphysis: A Biomechanical Study. *Arch. Orthop. Trauma Surg.* **2021**, *142*, 2235–2243. [CrossRef]
15. Moher, D.; Liberati, A.; Tetzlaff, J.; Altman, D.G. Preferred Reporting Items for Systematic Reviews and Meta-Analyses: The PRISMA Statement. *BMJ* **2009**, *339*, b2535. [CrossRef]
16. Moga, C.; Guo, B.; Schopflocher, D.; Harstall, C. *Development of a Quality Appraisal Tool for Case Series Studies Using a Modified Delphi Technique*; Institute of Health Economics: Edmonton, AB, Canada, 2012.
17. Coleman, B.D.; Khan, K.M.; Maffulli, N.; Cook, J.L.; Wark, J.D. Studies of Surgical Outcome after Patellar Tendinopathy: Clinical Significance of Methodological Deficiencies and Guidelines for Future Studies. *Scand. J. Med. Sci. Sports* **2000**, *10*, 2–11. [CrossRef]
18. Dewan, V.; Webb, M.S.L.; Prakash, D.; Malik, A.; Gella, S.; Kipps, C. When Does the Patella Dislocate? A Systematic Review of Biomechanical & Kinematic Studies. *J. Orthop.* **2020**, *20*, 70–77. [CrossRef]
19. Critical Appraisal Skills Programme CASP Cohort Study Checklist. Available online: http://docs.wixstatic.com/ugd/dded87_5ad0ece77a3f4fc9bcd3665a7d1fa91f.pdf (accessed on 14 April 2021).
20. Wilke, J.; Krause, F.; Niederer, D.; Engeroff, T.; Nürnberger, F.; Vogt, L.; Banzer, W. Appraising the Methodological Quality of Cadaveric Studies: Validation of the QUACS Scale. *J. Anat.* **2015**, *226*, 440–446. [CrossRef]
21. Higgins, J.P.T.; Thompson, S.G.; Deeks, J.J.; Altman, D.G. Measuring Inconsistency in Meta-Analyses. *BMJ* **2003**, *327*, 557–560. [CrossRef]
22. Chen, L.; Zhang, G.; Song, D.; Guo, X.; Yuan, W. A Comparison of Percutaneous Reduction and Screw Fixation versus Open Reduction and Plate Fixation of Traumatic Symphysis Pubis Diastasis. *Arch. Orthop. Trauma Surg.* **2012**, *132*, 265–270. [CrossRef]
23. Eakin, J.L.; Grewal, I.S.; Fene, E.S.; Sathy, A.K.; Starr, A.J. Percutaneous Screw Fixation of Pubic Symphysis Disruption: A Preliminary Report. *J. Clin. Orthop. Trauma* **2022**, *26*, 101806. [CrossRef] [PubMed]
24. Chan, A.C.K.; Chui, K.H.; Lee, K.B.; Li, W. Three-Dimensional Navigation-Guided Percutaneous Trans-Symphyseal Screw for Mechanically Unstable Pubic Symphysis Diastasis. *J. Orthop. Trauma Rehabil.* **2022**, *30*, 1–11. [CrossRef]
25. Cano-Luis, P.; Giráldez-Sanchez, M.A.; Martínez-Reina, J.; Serrano-Escalante, F.J.; Galleguillos-Rioboo, C.; Lázaro-Gonzálvez, A.; García-Rodríguez, J.; Navarro, A. Biomechanical Analysis of a New Minimally Invasive System for Osteosynthesis of Pubis Symphysis Disruption. *Injury* **2012**, *43*, 20–27. [CrossRef] [PubMed]
26. Gonzálvez, Á.L.; Reina, J.M.; Luis, P.C.; Baquero, J.J.; Fernández, J.S.; Sánchez, M.Á.G.; Lázaro Gonzálvez, Á.; Martínez Reina, J.; Cano Luis, P.; Jiménez Baquero, J.; et al. Is Cannulated-Screw Fixation an Alternative to Plate Osteosynthesis in Open Book Fractures? A Biomechanical Analysis. *Injury* **2016**, *47*, S72–S77. [CrossRef] [PubMed]
27. Sun, G.; Yin, C.; Liu, Z.; Wang, L.; Mu, W. Three-Dimensionally-Navigated Cross-Cannulated Screw Fixation for Traumatic Pubic Symphysis Diastasis: An Anatomical Study. *Acta Orthop. Traumatol. Turc.* **2016**, *50*, 214–221. [CrossRef]
28. Xu, P.; Wang, H.; Liu, Z.; Mu, W.; Xu, S.; Wang, L.; Chen, C.; Cavanaugh, J.M. An Evaluation of Three-Dimensional Image-Guided Technologies in Percutaneous Pelvic and Acetabular Lag Screw Placement. *J. Surg. Res.* **2013**, *185*, 338–346. [CrossRef]
29. Yao, F.; He, Y.; Qian, H.; Zhou, D.; Li, Q. Comparison of Biomechanical Characteristics and Pelvic Ring Stability Using Different Fixation Methods to Treat Pubic Symphysis Diastasis a Finite Element Study. *Medicine* **2015**, *94*, e2207. [CrossRef]
30. Yu, K.; Hong, J.; Sun, Y.; Shi, C.; Guo, X.; Zhou, D. Anatomical Measurement and Finite Element Study on Screw Channel Parameter in Percutaneous Fixation of Canulated Screw for Symphyseolysis. *Cell Biochem. Biophys.* **2015**, *71*, 1243–1248. [CrossRef]

31. Liu, L.; Fan, S.; Zeng, D.; Song, H.; Zeng, L.; Wen, X.; Jin, D. Identification of Safe Channels for Screws in the Anterior Pelvic Ring Fixation System. *J. Orthop. Surg. Res.* **2022**, *17*, 312. [CrossRef]
32. O'Neill, D.E.; Bradley, H.R.; Hull, B.; Pierce, W.; Grewal, I.S.; Starr, A.J.; Sathy, A.; Neill, D.E.O.; Bradley, H.R.; Hull, B.; et al. Percutaneous Screw Fixation of the Pubic Symphysis versus Plate Osteosynthesis: A Biomechanical Study. *OTA Int.* **2022**, *5*, e215. [CrossRef]
33. Majeed, S.A. Grading the Outcome of Pelvic Fractures. *J. Bone Joint Surg. Br.* **1989**, *71*, 304–306. [CrossRef]
34. Becker, I.; Woodley, S.J.; Stringer, M.D. The Adult Human Pubic Symphysis: A Systematic Review. *J. Anat.* **2010**, *217*, 475–487. [CrossRef]
35. Sagi, H.C.; Papp, S. Comparative Radiographic and Clinical Outcome of Two-Hole and Multi-Hole Symphyseal Plating. *J. Orthop. Trauma* **2008**, *22*, 373–378. [CrossRef]
36. Virkus, W.V.; Goldberg, S.H.; Lorenz, E.P. A Comparison of Compressive Force Generation by Plating and Intramedullary Nailing Techniques in a Transverse Diaphyseal Humerus Fracture Model. *J. Trauma* **2008**, *65*, 103–108. [CrossRef]

Journal of
Clinical Medicine

MDPI

Article

Demographics and Comorbidities of United States Service Members with Combat-Related Lower Extremity Limb Salvage

Stephen M. Goldman [1,2], Susan L. Eskridge [3], Sarah R. Franco [1,2] and Christopher L. Dearth [1,2,*]

1 Research & Surveillance Division, DoD-VA Extremity Trauma and Amputation Center of Excellence, 8901 Wisconsin Ave., Bethesda, MD 20889, USA
2 Department of Surgery, Uniformed Services University of the Health Sciences and Walter Reed National Military Medical Center, Bethesda, MD 20814, USA
3 Leidos, Reston, VA 20190, USA
* Correspondence: christopher.l.dearth.civ@health.mil; Tel.: +1-301-319-2461

Abstract: Introduction: This retrospective study describes the demographics and injury characteristics of a recently identified cohort of US Service members with combat-related lower extremity limb salvage (LS). Methods: US Service members with combat trauma were identified from the Expeditionary Medical Encounter Database and Military Health System Data Repository and stratified into primary amputation (PA), LS, and non-threatened limb trauma (NTLT) cohorts based on ICD-9 codes. Disparities in demographic factors and injury characteristics were investigated across cohorts and within the LS cohort based on limb retention outcome. Results: Cohort demographics varied by age but not by sex, branch, or rank. The mechanism of injury and injury characteristics were found to be different between the cohorts, with the LS cohort exhibiting more blast injuries and greater injury burden than their peers with NTLT. A sub-analysis of the LS population revealed more blast injuries and fewer gunshot wounds in those that underwent secondary amputation. Neither demographic factors nor total injury burden varied with limb retention outcome, despite slight disparities in AIS distribution within the LS cohort. Conclusions: In accordance with historic dogma, the LS population presents high injury severity. Demographics and injury characteristics are largely invariant with respect to limb retention outcomes, despite secondary amputation being moderately more prevalent in LS patients with blast-induced injuries. Further study of this population is necessary to better understand the factors that impact the outcomes of LS in the Military Health System.

Keywords: trauma; abbreviated injury scale; military medicine; wound and injuries; amputation; musculoskeletal system

1. Introduction

Extremity injuries constituted the majority of trauma experienced by United States Service members (SMs) during Operation Iraqi Freedom and Operation Enduring Freedom [1–3]. These types of injuries often involve multiple organ systems, adding complexity to their clinical care [4]. In many cases, the accumulated injuries pose a risk of limb loss, requiring a shared decision-making process between the patient and the clinical team to determine whether limb retention or immediate amputation is the preferred treatment strategy [5,6]. SMs who opt for limb retention often undergo multiple surgical procedures and intensive physical rehabilitation, collectively known as limb salvage (LS).

While the term "limb salvage" is commonly used, its precise definition has historically varied among providers. Consequently, conducting comprehensive epidemiological studies using large medical databases to assess the prevalence or incidence of LS in the context of lower extremity trauma has been challenging, and this population of SMs is understudied relative to other cohorts with readily identifiable medical codes (e.g., limb loss). As such, studies are often limited to studying a subset of limb salvage, as defined by either a narrow subset of injury types (e.g., Type III Gustilo Fractures [7], arterial injuries [8]) or a particular management plan (e.g., flap-based repair, vascular reconstruction) [9–12]. Subsequently, sample sizes are small, and interpretations are limited in scope.

This study aims to address this knowledge gap by utilizing a cohort of SMs with combat-related lower extremity (LE) LS, defined through a validated data-driven approach [13]. This study seeks to answer the following questions: (1) What are the demographic characteristics associated with the combat-related LS cohort? (2) What concomitant injuries are more frequently sustained by SMs who undergo LS? (3) Are there any correlated concomitant injuries that lead to secondary amputations?

2. Methods

2.1. Data Sources and Study Sample

This study was approved by the Naval Health Research Center (NHRC) Institutional Review Board and consisted of a retrospective database review of all combat-related injuries to lower extremities from 2004 to 2014 with an acute injury episode documented in the Expeditionary Medical Encounter Database (EMED; NHRC, San Diego, CA, USA) [14]. Inclusion criteria included the requirement of inpatient medical records within two years of the date of injury accessible within the Military Health System Data Repository (MDR). Exclusion criteria included a maximum lower extremity abbreviated injury scale (AIS) of one (i.e., minor trauma). Subsequently, an initial population of 4275 SMs with combat-related lower extremity trauma was identified. The initial population was then stratified into primary amputations (PA; i.e., amputation occurring $\leq$14 days after injury), non-threatened limb trauma (NTLT), and limb salvage (LS) cohorts using a combination of medical codes that has previously been reported to be significantly associated with limb salvage [13]. The identified LS cohort was further partitioned into those who went on to receive a secondary amputation (LS-SA, i.e., an amputation occurring $\geq$15 days after injury) and those who never underwent amputation (LS-NA). The PA and NTLT cohorts served as comparison groups.

2.2. Variables

Demographic variables, including age, sex, military branch, pay grade, the mechanism of injury, injury severity score (ISS), and maximum lower extremity abbreviated injury scale (AIS) were extracted from EMED records. The military branch was categorized as Army, Marine Corps, or other. Pay grade was categorized according to military rank: E1–E3, E4–E6, E7–E9, or Officer. Mechanisms of injury included blast, gunshot wound, or other. ISS was categorized based on severity mix as 1–4, 5–8, 9–15, 16–24, 25–49, or 50–75 [1].

Given the nature of combat-related trauma and the associated likelihood of injury to multiple body regions, especially in injury events due to explosions [2], the frequency of concomitant injuries was compared across cohorts. The concomitant injuries examined were selected a priori to include body regions and injury types that are characteristic of polytrauma and can influence recovery and rehabilitation following LS. Concomitant injuries were identified from initial injury coding from EMED using ICD-9-CM diagnosis codes (Table 1).

Table 1. Definition of co-occurring injuries.

Injury Description	ICD-9 Code
Fracture of skull	800–804.3
Fracture of spine and trunk	805–809.1
Fracture of upper limb	810–819.1
Intracranial injury; excludes skull fractures	850–854.1
Internal injury of chest, abdomen, and pelvis	860–869.1
Traumatic hemothorax/pneumothorax	860
Injury to heart/lung	861
Injury to other/unspec intrathoracic	862

Table 1. *Cont.*

Injury Description	ICD-9 Code
Injury to GI tract	863
Injury to liver	864
Injury to spleen	865
Injury to kidney	866
Injury to pelvic organs	867
Injury to intra-abdominal	868
Other internal	869
Open wounds on head, neck, and trunk	870–879.9
Open wounds on upper limb	880–887.7
Injury to blood vessels; excludes lower limb	900–903.9
Head	900
Thorax	901
Abdomen/pelvis	902
Upper limb	903
Injury to nerves and spinal cord; excludes LE	950–955.9
Injury to optic nerve	950
Injury to other cranial nerves	951
Spinal injury without bone injury	952
Injury to nerve roots/spinal plexus	953
Injury to other nerves of trunk	954
Injury to upper limb nerves	955
Burns	940–949.9

Note: Subordinate code descriptions are represented in italics.

2.3. Statistical Analysis

Categorical variables are displayed as counts along with their respective percentages, while continuous variables are presented as the mean and standard deviation (SD). To compare continuous variables, we conducted *t*-tests, and for categorical variables, we utilized chi-square tests, followed by post hoc Fisher's exact tests with Bonferroni correction, setting alpha at 0.05. All calculations were performed using IBM SPSS Statistics (Version 28.0.1.1, IBM Corp, Armonk, NY, USA).

3. Results

While there was a nominal difference (Table 2) in the age of the extremity trauma cohorts ($p = 0.008$), no differences were observed between groups with respect to sex ($p = 0.569$), branch of the military ($p = 0.348$), or pay grade ($p = 0.317$). The LS cohort is predominantly male (98.0%) with an average age of 25.6 ± 6.1 years. A total of 70.4% of the cohort is from the Army, while 26.6 belongs to the Marine Corps. The overwhelming majority of the cohort comes from the enlisted ranks. No difference in age, sex, branch, or pay grade was observed for the LS subgroups associated with limb retention outcome (Table 3). The mechanism of injury was found to be different ($\chi^2 = 356.1$, 6 DF, $p < 0.001$) between the cohorts, with the PA cohort exhibiting the highest prevalence of blast injuries (95.5%) and LS (79.3%) and NTLT (64.9%) exhibiting lower rates in a stepwise fashion. Subsequently, gunshot wounds (GSWs) followed the opposite pattern, with NTLT exhibiting the highest prevalence (31.3%), followed by LS (16.9%) and PA (2.0%). Further analysis of the LS subgroups revealed that the LS-SA cohort experienced a higher prevalence of blast injuries (89.2%) and a lower prevalence of GSWs (7.1%) relative to the LS-NA cohort (blast 77.8%, GSW 18.4%).

Injury severity score (ISS) also varied across the LE trauma cohorts both with respect to the population mean ($p < 0.001$) and distribution ($p < 0.001$). The mean ISS for the LS cohort was higher than those with NTLT ($p < 0.001$) but lower than their peers with PA ($p < 0.001$). When binned according to severity mix [15], it was found that SMs belonging to the LS cohort were more likely to have an ISS in the range of 4–8 or 9–15 than their peers with PA and less likely to fall into severity mixes of 16–24 or 25–49. Compared with the

NTLT cohort, the LS cohort exhibited an ISS distribution skewed toward a higher severity mix. Notably, the NTLT cohort exhibited a higher prevalence of ISS scores in the 4–8 range (37.0% vs. 27.1%, $p < 0.001$), while the LS cohort exhibited a higher prevalence of ISS scores in the 9–15 range. No differences between groups were observed for higher-scoring bins. No difference in the mean ISS ($p = 0.707$) or severity mix was observed between the LS subgroups.

Table 2. Demographics and injury characteristics by cohort designation.

Classifiers	PA N = 885	LS N = 2018	NTLT N = 1372	Adjusted p-Values		
				χ^2 Test or ANOVA	Fisher's Exact	
					PA vs. LS	LS vs. NTLT
Age (mean ± SD)	24.9 ± 5.0	25.6 ± 6.1	25.4 ± 5.9	**0.008**	>0.999	>0.999
Male (n (%))	869 (98.2)	1977 (98.0)	1339 (97.6)	0.569		
Branch (n (%))				0.348		
Army	591 (66.8)	1421 (70.4)	942 (68.7)			
Marine Corps	260 (29.4)	536 (26.6)	386 (28.1)			
Other	34 (3.8)	61 (3.0)	44 (3.2)			
Pay grade (n (%)) †				0.317		
E1–E3	261 (29.5)	562 (27.8)	386 (28.1)			
E4–E6	519 (58.6)	1076 (53.4)	762 (53.6)			
E7–E9	34 (3.8)	102 (5.0)	77 (5.6)			
Officer	67 (7.6)	126 (6.2)	77 (5.6)			
Mechanism of injury (n (%))				**<0.001**		
Blast	845 (95.5)	1601 (79.3)	891 (64.9)	**<0.001**	**<0.001**	**<0.001**
Gunshot wound	18 (2.0)	341 (16.9)	429 (31.3)	**<0.001**	**<0.001**	**<0.001**
Other	22 (2.5)	76 (3.8)	52 (3.8)	0.178		
ISS (mean ± SD)	20.1 ± 10.7	12.6 ± 8.8	11.8 ± 8.9	**<0.001**	**<0.001**	**<0.001**
ISS categories (n (%))				**<0.001**		
1–3	--	--	--	--	--	--
4–8	1055 (31.1)	547 (27.1)	508 (37.0)	**<0.001**	**<0.001**	**<0.001**
9–15	1531 (45.2)	979 (48.5)	552 (40.2)	**<0.001**	**<0.001**	**<0.001**
16–24	500 (14.7)	315 (15.6)	185 (13.5)	**<0.001**	**<0.001**	0.254
25–49	277 (8.2)	158 (7.8)	119 (8.7)	**<0.001**	**<0.001**	0.545
50–75	27 (0.8)	19 (0.9)	8 (0.6)	**0.038**	0.161	0.545
Max lower extremity AIS (n (%))				**<0.001**		
1	--	--	--	--	--	--
2	1708 (50.4)	885 (43.9)	823 (60.0)	**<0.001**	**<0.001**	**<0.001**
3	1531 (45.2)	1026 (50.8)	505 (36.8)	**<0.001**	0.113	**<0.001**
4	113 (3.3)	89 (4.4)	24 (1.7)	**<0.001**	**<0.001**	**<0.001**
5	38 (1.1)	18 (0.9)	20 (1.5)	**<0.001**	**<0.001**	0.136
Polytrauma (n (%)) *	269 (30.4)	302 (15.0)	212 (15.4)	**<0.001**	**<0.001**	0.697

Note: † Percent does not add up to zero due to missing data. * Polytrauma is defined as two AIS regions > 2. Statistically significant findings are indicated by bolded p-values. Subordinate classifiers are represented by italics.

Table 3. Demographics and injury characteristics of limb salvage population by outcome.

Classifiers	LS-SA n = 269	LS-NA n = 1749	Adjusted p-Values
Age (mean (SD))	24.8 ± 5.1	25.7 ± 6.2	0.187
Male (n (%))	266 (98.9)	1711 (97.8)	1.000
Branch (n (%))			
Army	176 (65.4)	1245 (71.2)	0.770

Table 3. *Cont.*

Classifiers	LS-SA n = 269	LS-NA n = 1749	Adjusted *p*-Values
Marine Corps	81 (30.1)	455 (26.0)	0.981
Other	12 (4.5)	49 (2.8)	0.989
Pay grade (n (%)) †			
E1–E3	90 (33.5)	472 (27.0)	0.548
E4–E6	141 (52.4)	935 (53.5)	1.000
E7–E9	12 (4.5)	90 (5.2)	1.000
Officer	22 (8.2)	104 (5.9)	0.988
Mechanism of injury (n (%))			
Blast	**240 (89.2)**	**1361 (77.8)**	**<0.001**
Gunshot wound	**19 (7.1)**	**322 (18.4)**	**<0.001**
Other	10 (3.7)	66 (3.8)	1.000
ISS (mean (SD))	13.8 ± 10.4	12.5 ± 8.5	0.707
ISS categories (n (%))			
1–4	0	0	--
5–8	59 (21.9)	488 (27.9)	0.661
9–15	142 (52.8)	837 (47.9)	0.962
16–24	44 (16.4)	271 (15.5)	1.000
25–49	17 (6.3)	141 (8.0)	1.000
50–75	7 (2.6)	12 (0.7)	0.169
Max lower extremity AIS (n (%))			
1	0	0	--
2	**92 (34.2)**	**793 (45.3)**	**0.014**
3	**162 (60.2)**	**864 (49.4)**	**0.023**
4	9 (3.3)	80 (4.6)	1.000
5	6 (2.2)	12 (0.7)	0.432

Note: † Indicates that percentages do not add up to 100 due to missing data. Statistically significant findings are indicated by bolding. Subordinate classifiers are represented by italics.

The distribution of the maximum LE AIS score was disparate between the LE trauma cohorts (χ^2 = 1359, 6 DF, $p < 0.001$). While a maximum LE AIS score of two was most prevalent for the NTLT cohort, post hoc Fisher's exact tests revealed that SMs from the LS cohort were more likely to have a maximum LE AIS of three (50.8% > 36.8%, $p < 0.001$) or four (4.4% > 1.7%, $p < 0.001$) relative to NTLT but less likely to have a maximum LE AIS score of four (29.3% > 4.4%, $p < 0.001$) or five (16.9% > 0.9%, $p < 0.001$) than the PA cohort. No difference was observed between LS and NTLT for maximum LE AIS scores of five. Among the LS cohorts, SMs from the LS-SA cohort were found to be less likely to have a maximum LE AIS score of two (34.2% < 45.3%, $p = 0.014$) and more likely to have a maximum LE AIS score of three (60.2% > 49.4%, $p = 0.023$) than the LS-NA cohort. No difference was observed between the two LS cohorts for maximum LE AIS scores of four or five. The prevalence of polytrauma also varied across cohorts, with PA exhibiting greater representation than LS (30.4% > 15.0%, $p < 0.001$). No difference in the prevalence of polytrauma was observed between LS and NTLT or between LS subgroups.

Analysis of co-occurring injuries revealed each of the injury patterns studied was disparately observed within the extremity trauma cohorts (Table 4). Relative to NTLT, the LS cohort exhibited a greater rate of fracture of the skull (Fisher's Exact, $p = 0.010$) and lower rates of fracture of the spine and trunk (Fisher's Exact, $p < 0.001$) and internal injury of the chest, abdomen, and pelvis ($p = 0.010$). Relative to PA, the LS cohort exhibited lower rates of internal injuries of the chest, abdomen, and pelvis ($p < 0.001$), open wounds on the head, neck, and trunk ($p < 0.001$), open wounds on the upper limbs ($p < 0.001$), injuries to blood vessels ($p < 0.001$), injuries to nerves and the spinal cord ($p < 0.010$), and burns ($p = 0.030$). No disparities in co-occurring injuries were observed between the LS subgroups (Table 5).

Table 4. Co-occurring injuries by lower extremity trauma cohort designation.

Injuries	PA N = 885		LS N = 2018		NTLT N = 1372		χ^2 Test	Fisher's Exact Test Adjusted *p*-Value	
	f	%	*f*	%	*f*	%	*p*-Value	PA vs. LS	LS vs. NTLT
Fracture of skull	98	11.1	225	11.1	107	7.8	0.003	>0.999	0.010
Fracture of spine and trunk	165	18.6	375	18.6	359	26.2	<0.001	>0.999	<0.001
Fracture of upper limb	321	36.3	406	20.1	232	16.9	<0.001	<0.001	0.183
Intracranial injury; excludes skull fractures	317	35.8	655	32.5	399	29.1	0.003	0.566	0.321
Internal injury of chest, abdomen, and pelvis	224	25.3	327	16.2	287	20.9	<0.001	<0.001	0.010
Open wounds on head, neck, and trunk	538	60.8	894	44.3	590	43.0	<0.001	<0.001	0.998
Open wounds on upper limb	493	55.7	1215	60.2	870	63.4	<0.001	<0.001	1.000
Injury to blood vessels; excludes LE	91	10.3	560	27.7	116	8.4	<0.001	<0.001	0.757
Injury to nerves and spinal cord; excludes LE	110	12.4	171	8.5	143	10.3	0.003	0.010	0.467
Burns	117	13.2	190	9.4	128	9.3	0.003	0.030	1.000

Note: Frequencies represent the number of service members with at least one of the indicated diagnoses.

Table 5. Co-occurring injuries by lower extremity trauma cohort designation.

Injuries	LS-SA		LS-NA N = 1749		Fisher's Exact Test
	f	%	*f*	%	*p*-Value
Fracture of skull	32	11.9	193	11.0	>0.999
Fracture of spine and trunk	58	21.6	317	18.1	0.861
Fracture of upper limb	57	21.2	349	19.9	>0.999
Intracranial injury; excludes skull fractures	99	36.8	556	31.8	0.681
Internal injury of chest, abdomen, and pelvis	52	19.3	275	15.7	0.814
Open wounds on head, neck, and trunk	119	44.2	775	44.3	>0.999
Open wounds on upper limb	71	26.4	559	32.0	0.551
Injury to blood vessels; excludes LE	15	5.6	90	5.1	>0.999
Injury to nerves and spinal cord; excludes LE	22	8.2	149	8.5	>0.999
Burns	25	9.3	165	9.4	>0.999

Note: Frequencies represent the number of service members with at least one of the indicated diagnoses.

4. Discussion

The observations reported herein represent the demographic profile and concomitant injuries of a cohort of SMs who underwent combat-related LS, and the subgroups within it based on penultimate limb retention outcome. In accordance with the prior literature [16], the LS cohort was characterized by more severely injured extremities relative to the NTLT comparison group and a high degree of polytrauma, yet this cohort had less severe injuries and a lower degree of polytrauma relative to PA. This is likely explained by the relative prevalence of blast injuries among the extremity trauma cohorts, as it is well established that polytrauma is commonly seen as a result of explosive mechanisms [17] due to blast-related primary (results from blast wave through the body), secondary (results from flying debris), tertiary (results from being thrown by the blast), and quaternary (all other explosion-related injuries) injuries [18]. Among the concomitant injuries more prevalent within the LS population, vascular injuries affecting body regions exclusive of the lower extremities were found to exhibit the most disparate frequency. This disparity is also likely explained by the prevalence of the blast mechanism of injury in this group, as it has previously been reported that explosive munitions were commonly associated with penetrating vascular injury [19,20].

The NTLT cohort had a higher prevalence of internal injury of the chest, abdomen, and pelvis compared to the LS cohort (16.2% vs. 20.9%; $p = 0.010$). This observation has multiple plausible explanations. First, the disparity may be linked to the fact that gunshot wounds (GSWs) were the predominant mechanism of injury among the NTLT cohort. Evidence in the literature from civilian public mass shootings suggests a strong relationship between the number of GSWs and the number of fatal organ injuries. Moreover, the location of the GSW varied by body area, with the chest/upper back and extremities both exhibiting > 1 GSW per victim, representing a significantly higher prevalence than the head and neck regions [21]. Furthermore, it was also noted that the location of the fatal wound occurring in the extremity in these cases was rare. If we apply this knowledge from the civilian world to a military context, wherein the usage of body armor has been associated with a sizeable reduction in the number of fatal thoracic injuries, irrespective of the mechanism of injury, incurred during conflict situations [22,23], it is plausible that the higher prevalence of internal thoracic injuries observed within the NTLT cohort could be associated with behind armor blunt trauma (BABT), which is succinctly defined as a non-penetrating thoracic injury due to the rapid deformation of body armor impacted by a high-energy projectile [24]. Based on the dependence of BABT on energy transfer, it is unlikely that such injuries would occur as frequently via explosive mechanisms, as the kinetic energy of the blast fragments can be substantially lower than bullets owing to the size and spread of the projectiles as well as the distance of the victim from the explosion. Further regional analysis of non-fatal ballistic wounding patterns among combat-injured SMs is necessary to support this conjecture.

Further analysis of the LS cohort revealed that individuals who entered the LS treatment pathway but ultimately opted for or required treatment with amputation (i.e., secondary amputation, LS-SA) exhibited higher LE AIS scores of 3, whereas the cohort that did not experience limb loss (i.e., LS-NA) more often exhibited a maximum LE AIS score of 2. While it is possible, even likely, that the disparities in limb retention outcomes within the LS cohort are at least partially explained by the observed disparities in the wounding mechanism and resultant local injury burden between LS-SA and LS-NA, it is also plausible that there are differences in pathology and/or clinical care that have not yet been elucidated and require further study in order to move toward understanding what factors are correlated with or predictive of limb retention outcomes of a limb salvage patient.

5. Limitations

These results presented herein suggest that the combat-related LS population is indicative of a greater portion of highly complex cases than NTLT, as determined by AIS and ISS. However, importantly, there are inherent limitations to making inferences based on AIS and ISS. Specifically, ISS does not account for multiple injuries to the same body part [25]. Despite past modifications made to AIS to make it more applicable to combat injuries (i.e., AIS-2005-Military and AIS-2008-Military), significant drawbacks in using this scoring system to adequately address the complexity of injuries suffered by SMs remain [26]. This study addressed the limitations of AIS, in part, by characterizing the concomitant injuries sustained by SMs with LS.

Another limitation of this study is that it does not report specifics on the proximity of the associated vascular injuries to the lower extremity, nor are there details of the operative techniques used to repair the injured vessels (e.g., autologous grafts, bypass, and ligation).

Furthermore, details on total limb ischemia time (if any) and interval to reperfusion, both of which are directly correlated with adverse events, are not reported, as they were outside of the scope of this study but warrant future investigation.

Finally, this study only investigated one surgical outcome of LS, namely limb retention. Future efforts will more comprehensively define this LS cohort in terms of rates of acquired secondary musculoskeletal health conditions and return to duty, as well as evaluate healthcare utilization patterns.

6. Conclusions

The aim of this study was to examine the demographics and associated injuries in a group of service members who underwent limb salvage procedures. As expected, the LS group had less severe injuries compared to the primary amputation group, but their injuries were more serious than those in the non-threatening limb trauma group. This difference is likely due to the higher incidence of blast-induced injuries in the cohorts. Within the LS subgroups, despite similar demographic characteristics, there were variations in the mechanisms of injury and injury severity. Those who ultimately required secondary amputation had higher rates of blast injuries and higher maximum lower extremity injury scores (AIS). This observation emphasizes the importance of considering injury mechanisms and severity when distinguishing LS from other SM groups with extremity injuries. Furthermore, our findings highlight the necessity for further research on the LS population to gain a better understanding of the factors that impact patient outcomes so as to (1) enhance tools for clinical decision making and (2) identify capability gaps in the development of next-generation diagnostics and therapies.

Author Contributions: Conceptualization: S.M.G., S.L.E. and C.L.D.; data curation: S.M.G., S.L.E., S.R.F. and C.L.D.; formal analysis: S.M.G., S.L.E., S.R.F. and C.L.D.; writing—original draft: S.M.G.; writing—review and editing: S.M.G., S.L.E., S.R.F. and C.L.D. All authors have read and agreed to the published version of the manuscript.

Funding: Support for this study was provided by the DoD-VA Extremity Trauma and Amputation Center of Excellence (Award # HU00012020038).

Institutional Review Board Statement: The study was conducted in accordance with the Declaration of Helsinki was and approved by the Institutional Review Board of the Naval Health Research Center. All methods were performed in accordance with the relevant guidelines and regulations.

Informed Consent Statement: This retrospective study was conducted using de-identified data, ensuring the privacy and confidentiality of all individuals involved. As such, informed consent was not required or obtained from the subjects of this study, as no personally identifiable information was used.

Data Availability Statement: All data supporting the findings of this study are available within the paper.

Conflicts of Interest: The opinions or assertions contained herein are the private ones of the author/speaker and are not to be construed as official or reflecting the views of the Department of Defense, the Uniformed Services University of the Health Sciences or any other agency of the U.S. Government. The authors have no conflict of interest to declare.

References

1. Belmont, P.J., Jr.; Goodman, G.P.; Zacchilli, M.; Posner, M.; Evans, C.; Owens, B.D. Incidence and Epidemiology of Combat Injuries Sustained During "The Surge" Portion of Operation Iraqi Freedom by a U.S. Army Brigade Combat Team. *J. Trauma Acute Care Surg.* **2010**, *68*, 204–210. [CrossRef] [PubMed]
2. Owens, B.D.; Kragh, J.F.; Wenke, J.C.; Macaitis, J.; Wade, C.E.; Holcomb, J.B. Combat wounds in operation Iraqi Freedom and operation Enduring Freedom. *J. Trauma* **2008**, *64*, 295–299. [CrossRef] [PubMed]
3. Eskridge, S.L.; Macera, C.A.; Galarneau, M.R.; Holbrook, T.L.; Woodruff, S.I.; MacGregor, A.J.; Morton, D.J.; Shaffer, R.A. Injuries from combat explosions in Iraq: Injury type, location, and severity. *Injury* **2012**, *43*, 1678–1682. [CrossRef] [PubMed]
4. McDonald, S.J.; Sun, M.; Agoston, D.V.; Shultz, S.R. The effect of concomitant peripheral injury on traumatic brain injury pathobiology and outcome. *J. Neuroinflamm.* **2016**, *13*, 90. [CrossRef]

5. Beeharry, M.W.; Walden-Smith, T.; Moqeem, K. Limb Salvage vs. Amputation: Factors Influencing the Decision-Making Process and Outcomes for Mangled Extremity Injuries. *Cureus* **2022**, *14*, e30817. [CrossRef]
6. Sharrock, M. The mangled extremity: Assessment, decision making and outcomes. *Acta Orthop. Belg.* **2021**, *87*, 755–760. [CrossRef]
7. Ozmen, E.; Balci, H.I.; Salduz, A.; Eralp, İ.L. Limb salvage results of Gustilo IIIC fractures of the lower extremity. *Acta Orthop. Belg.* **2022**, *88*, 569–573. [CrossRef]
8. Urrechaga, E.; Jabori, S.; Kang, N.; Kenel-Pierre, S.; Lopez, A.; Rattan, R.; Rey, J.; Bornak, A. Traumatic Lower Extremity Vascular Injuries and Limb Salvage in a Civilian Urban Trauma Center. *Ann. Vasc. Surg.* **2022**, *82*, 30–40. [CrossRef]
9. Casey, K.; Sabino, J.; Weiss, J.S.; Kumar, A.; Valerio, I. Limb salvage after vascular reconstruction followed by tissue transfer during the Global War on Terror. *J. Vasc. Surg.* **2015**, *61*, 734–740. [CrossRef]
10. Shastov, A.; Mikhailov, A.; Kliushin, N.; Malkova, T. Limb salvage and functional recovery in infected nonunion of the distal tibia treated with the Ilizarov techniques. *J. Clin. Orthop. Trauma* **2023**, *44*, 102255. [CrossRef]
11. Prasad, M.; Kaul, R.; Thakur, K.; Gupta, T.D.; Shakya, A.R. Efficacious Enactment of Ilizarov for Mangled Forearm: A Case Report on Our Resolution for the Revitalization of a "Nearly Lost Limb". *J. Orthop. Case Rep.* **2023**, *13*, 122–126. [CrossRef] [PubMed]
12. Tropf, J.G.; Hoyt, B.W.; Walsh, S.A.; Gibson, J.A.; Polfer, E.M.; Souza, J.M.; Potter, B.K. Long-Term Health Outcomes of Limb Salvage Compared with Amputation for Combat-Related Trauma. *J. Bone Jt. Surg.* **2023**. [CrossRef] [PubMed]
13. Goldman, S.M.; Eskridge, S.L.; Franco, S.R.; Souza, J.M.; Tintle, S.M.; Dowd, T.C.; Alderete, J.; Potter, B.K.; Dearth, C.L. A Data-Driven Method to Discriminate Limb Salvage from Other Combat-Related Extremity Trauma. *J. Clin. Med.* **2023**, *12*, 6357. [CrossRef] [PubMed]
14. Galarneau, M.R.; Hancock, W.C.; Konoske, P.; Melcer, T.; Vickers, R.R.; Walker, G.J.; Zouris, J.M. The Navy-Marine Corps Combat Trauma Registry. *Mil. Med.* **2006**, *171*, 691–697. [CrossRef] [PubMed]
15. Copes, W.S.; Champion, H.R.; Sacco, W.J.; Lawnick, M.M.; Keast, S.L.; Bain, L.W. The Injury Severity Score revisited. *J. Trauma* **1988**, *28*, 69–77. [CrossRef] [PubMed]
16. Bosse, M.J.; MacKenzie, E.J.; Kellam, J.F.; Burgess, A.R.; Webb, L.X.; Swiontkowski, M.F.; Sanders, R.W.; Jones, A.L.; McAndrew, M.P.; Patterson, B.M.; et al. An Analysis of Outcomes of Reconstruction or Amputation after Leg-Threatening Injuries. *N. Engl. J. Med.* **2002**, *347*, 1924–1931. [CrossRef]
17. Vuoncino, M.; Hoo, A.J.S.; Patel, J.A.; White, P.W.; Rasmussen, T.E.; White, J.M. Epidemiology of Upper Extremity Vascular Injury in Contemporary Combat. *Ann. Vasc. Surg.* **2020**, *62*, 98–103. [CrossRef]
18. Jorolemon, M.R.; Lopez, R.A.; Krywko, D.M. Blast Injuries. In *StatPearls*; StatPearls Publishing: Treasure Island, FL, USA, 2019.
19. Peck, M.A.; Clouse, W.D.; Cox, M.W.; Bowser, A.N.; Eliason, J.L.; Jenkins, D.H.; Smith, D.L.; Rasmussen, T.E. The complete management of extremity vascular injury in a local population: A wartime report from the 332nd Expeditionary Medical Group/Air Force Theater Hospital, Balad Air Base, Iraq. *J. Vasc. Surg.* **2007**, *45*, 1197–1204; discussion 1204–1205. [CrossRef]
20. Sohn, V.Y.; Arthurs, Z.M.; Herbert, G.S.; Beekley, A.C.; Sebesta, J.A. Demographics, treatment, and early outcomes in penetrating vascular combat trauma. *Arch. Surg.* **2008**, *143*, 783–787. [CrossRef]
21. Sarani, B.; Hendrix, C.; Matecki, M.; Estroff, J.; Amdur, R.L.; Robinson, B.R.; Shapiro, G.; Gondek, S.; Mitchell, R.; Smith, E.R. Wounding Patterns Based on Firearm Type in Civilian Public Mass Shootings in the United States. *J. Am. Coll. Surg.* **2019**, *228*, 228–234. [CrossRef]
22. Mabry, R.L.; Holcomb, J.B.; Baker, A.M.; Cloonan, C.C.; Uhorchak, J.M.; Perkins, D.E.; Canfield, A.J.; Hagmann, J.H. United States Army Rangers in Somalia: An analysis of combat casualties on an urban battlefield. *J. Trauma* **2000**, *49*, 515–528; discussion 528–529. [CrossRef]
23. Masini, B.D.; Waterman, S.M.; Wenke, J.C.; Owens, B.D.; Hsu, J.R.; Ficke, J.R. Resource utilization and disability outcome assessment of combat casualties from Operation Iraqi Freedom and Operation Enduring Freedom. *J. Orthop. Trauma* **2009**, *23*, 261–266. [CrossRef] [PubMed]
24. Cannon, L. Behind armour blunt trauma--an emerging problem. *J. R. Army Med. Corps* **2001**, *147*, 87–96. [CrossRef] [PubMed]
25. Wang, M.D.; Fan, W.H.; Qiu, W.S.; Zhang, Z.L.; Mo, Y.N.; Qiu, F. The exponential function transforms the Abbreviated Injury Scale, which both improves accuracy and simplifies scoring. *Eur. J. Trauma Emerg. Surg.* **2014**, *40*, 287–294. [CrossRef]
26. Lawnick, M.M.; Champion, H.R.; Gennarelli, T.; Galarneau, M.R.; D'Souza, E.; Vickers, R.R.; Wing, V.; Eastridge, B.J.; Young, L.A.; Dye, J.; et al. Combat injury coding: A review and reconfiguration. *J. Trauma Acute Care Surg.* **2013**, *75*, 573–581. [CrossRef] [PubMed]

Journal of
Clinical Medicine

MDPI

Article

Epidemiological Analysis of Traumatic Compartment Syndromes in Germany

Philipp Herrmann *, Annette Eidmann, Felix Hochberger, Tizian Heinz, Dominik Rak, Manuel Weißenberger, Maximilian Rudert and Ioannis Stratos

Department of Orthopaedic Surgery, Koenig-Ludwig-Haus, Julius-Maximilians University Wuerzburg, Brettreichstrasse 11, 97074 Wuerzburg, Germany; i-stratos.klh@uni-wuerzburg.de (I.S.)
* Correspondence: philipp.herrmann@klh.de

Abstract: Background: Traumatic compartment syndrome is a critical condition that can lead to severe, lifelong disability. **Methods**: This retrospective study analyzed hospital billing data from 2015 to 2022, provided by the Federal Statistical Office of Germany, to examine the demographics and trends of traumatic compartment syndrome in Germany. The analysis included cases coded with ICD-10 codes T79.60 to T79.69 and any therapeutic OPS code starting with 5–79, focusing on diagnosis year, gender, ICD-10 code, and patient age. **Results**: The results showed that out of 13,305 cases, the majority were in the lower leg (44.4%), with males having a significantly higher incidence than females (2.3:1 ratio). A bimodal age distribution was observed, with peaks at 22–23 and 55 years. A notable annual decline of 43.87 cases in compartment syndrome was observed, with significant decreases across different genders and age groups, particularly in males under 40 (23.68 cases per year) and in the "foot" and "lower leg" categories (16.67 and 32.87 cases per year, respectively). **Conclusions**: The study highlights a declining trend in traumatic CS cases in Germany, with distinct demographic patterns. Through these findings, hospitals can adjust their therapeutic regimens, and it could increase awareness among healthcare professionals about this disease.

Keywords: traumatic compartment syndrome; demographics; Germany; billing data; epidemiological trends; healthcare data analysis

1. Introduction

Compartment syndrome (CS) is a severe and potentially limb-threatening medical condition, most commonly arising following traumatic injuries. The causes of CS can be divided into traumatic and non-traumatic. Epidemiological studies have well established that fractures are the most common cause of traumatic compartment syndromes, accounting for about 69–75% of all cases [1–3]. Nevertheless, traumatic CS can also be triggered by other diverse factors, including soft tissue injuries, vascular injuries, penetrating trauma, or severe thermal burns [4–6].

Nontraumatic causes of CS occur less frequently but can be attributed to a broad spectrum of conditions. Disturbances in blood coagulation, resulting from anticoagulation therapy or coagulation disorders, have been identified as contributors to non-traumatic CS [7]. Furthermore, nephrotic syndrome, revascularization procedures or treatments, or Group A streptococcus infections of muscles are non-traumatic causes of CS [8–10]. The pathophysiology of CS is characterized by increased pressure within a closed anatomical space, known as a compartment, leading to compromised blood flow and tissue perfusion. The resulting osmotic imbalance exacerbates intracellular edema, ultimately leading to necrosis. Consequently, this triggers the release of inflammatory substances in the affected area, further increasing tissue swelling and pressure within the compartment [11]. Early diagnosis and rapid surgical decompression are essential to prevent irreversible damage. It is well established that the treatment of CS is a fasciotomy of all involved compartments [12].

Adjunctive treatments include removing all constrictive dressings, elevating the affected limb, maintaining normotensive blood pressure, and providing oxygen supplementation. The diagnosis of CS and the decision for surgical intervention remain challenging. The primary element in diagnosing CS continues to be clinical assessment. An initial indication of CS often involves experiencing pain that is out of proportion and a heightened need for analgesics [13]. As the condition progresses, neurovascular symptoms arise due to prolonged ischemia, manifesting as pallor, pulselessness, paralysis, and paresthesia [14]. In cases where a compartment syndrome is clinically suspected, particularly in unconscious patients where diagnosis proves challenging, measuring intercompartmental pressure serves as a valuable tool to confirm the diagnosis.

Compartment syndromes may occur as a chronic or acute syndrome. The acute compartment syndrome is a surgical emergency with potentially devastating consequences. Untreated acute CS can result in necrosis, infection, paralysis, and limb amputation [15]. A recent study showed that only 69.2% of patients returned to their initial work [16]. This highlights the socioeconomic impact of CS and the significance of early diagnosis and accurate treatment. Numerous studies in the literature focus on the diagnosis and management of CS, with a particular emphasis on isolated body regions.

To date, there is a lack of literature detailing the prevalence of traumatic CS. Furthermore, research has not been conducted to identify which anatomical regions are most affected by CS. Moreover, a significant gap exists in the literature concerning comprehensive analyses encompassing trends and demographic characteristics associated with traumatic CS with simultaneous osteosyntheses in Germany. Our research aimed to fill this gap by examining cases of traumatic compartment syndrome that were treated concurrently with osteosynthetic procedures. The objective of our study was to investigate the demographics and overall trends in Germany.

2. Materials and Methods

2.1. Data Source and Data Structure

The Hospital billing data for patients with fracture- or luxation-associated compartment syndromes, who simultaneously received osteosynthetic treatment, were obtained from the Federal Statistical Office of Germany for the years 2015 to 2022. For the purpose of this study, we defined traumatic compartment syndrome as a coded compartment syndrome with a simultaneous coded osteosynthesis upon fracture or dislocation during the same hospital stay. The data included the number of patients diagnosed with a compartment syndrome and those undergoing reposition of a fracture or dislocation with osteosynthesis during the same hospital stay. To identify these patients, billing cases were searched for a diagnosis code (International Statistical Classification of Diseases and Related Health Problems-10 code) from T79.60 to T79.69 (indicating any traumatic compartment syndrome) combined with any therapeutic code (Operation and Procedure Classification System code) that starts with 5–79 (representing any open or closed reposition of a fracture or luxation using implants). The OPS Code is a classification system used in Germany to code medical procedures and interventions. The data output was provided to our group by an employee of the Federal Statistical Office of Germany following specific instructions. It included the year of diagnosis (2015–2022), gender (male and female), the ICD-10 code (T79.60 to T79.69), and patient age (grouped in 5-year intervals). The data were presented in a grouped format and can be downloaded from the URL https://github.com/ioannis-stratos/compartment (generated and accessed on 7 January 2024).

2.2. Data Processing

This dataset was provided in a wide format. For further analysis, it was transformed from a wide format to a long format using R (version 2023.12.0, R-Studio; Boston, MA, USA) and the 'reshape2' library. Subgroup analysis was performed using the ICD-10 codes T79.60 (compartment syndrome of the upper extremities; "upper extremity group"), T79.61 (compartment syndrome of the hip and thigh; "hip and thigh group"), T79.62 (compartment syndrome of the lower leg; "lower leg group"), T79.63 (compartment syndrome of the foot; "foot group"), and T79.68 and T79.69 (compartment syndrome of other or unspecified localizations; "unspecified group"). Further subgroup analysis included gender, year of diagnosis, and patient age (grouped as "≥40 years" and "<40 years"). These subgroups were calculated and analyzed in tables using Tableau Desktop (version 2023.3, Tableau Software, Seattle, WA, USA).

2.3. Statistical Analysis

Using GraphPad Prism (version 10.1.1; GraphPad Software; San Diego, CA, USA), linear regression analyses were performed and diagrams generated. Linear regression analysis is a statistical method used to understand the relationship between a dependent variable and one or more independent variables. The F-test was used to determine if the overall significance of the linear regression model was significantly different from zero. For nonlinear regression analysis, Lorentzian distributions, a continuous probability distribution, were employed. The χ^2-test was applied to assess differences in group distributions. The significance level was set at $p \leq 0.05$ for the statistical analyses.

3. Results

During the period from 2015 to 2022, we reviewed a total of 13,305 cases of traumatic compartment syndromes. Of these, 61% manifested in the lower extremities and 11% in the upper extremities. A significant portion of cases lacked precise localization classification (25.2%). Most traumatic compartment syndromes occurred in males (4092 cases in females vs. 9213 in males), resulting in a female to male ratio 1:2.3 (Table 1). Subgroup analysis, differentiating between younger patients (<40 years) and older patients (≥40 years), revealed that most younger patients were male (male to female ratio of 5.1:1). In contrast, the older age group showed an increased proportion of females (male to female ratio of 1.7:1) (Figure 1). The distribution of males and females within younger and older patients was equal in the group "foot". For all other localizations (unspecified, lower leg, hip and thigh, upper extremities), the male to female ratio decreased significantly in patients above 40 years of age (Figure 1).

Table 1. Summary of total numbers of traumatic compartment syndromes between 2015 and 2022, categorized by localization (foot, upper extremity, hip and thigh, lower leg, and unspecific location) and patient sex (male and female).

	Foot	Upper Extremity	Hip and Thigh	Lower Leg	Unspecified Location	Total
Male patients (% of total)	936 10.2%	952 10.3%	655 7.1%	4616 50.1%	2054 22.3%	9213 100%
Female patients (% of total)	260 6.4%	446 10.9%	336 8.2%	1755 42.9%	1295 31.6%	4092 100%
Sum male & female (% of total)	1196 9.0%	1398 10.5%	991 7.4%	5911 44.4%	3349 25.2%	13,305 100%
Ratio male:female	3.6	2.1	1.9	2.6	1.6	2.3

In most localizations, the age distribution shows a bimodal trend. The initial peak occurs at the age of 22 and 23, with distinct peaks at different sites: the "foot" at 21.88 years, the "lower leg" at 23.32 years, and the "hip and thigh" at 22.84 years. The second peak is observed at 55 years, with the "foot" peaking at 55.58 years and the "lower leg" at 55.49 years. However, for the "hip and thigh," the second peak is considerably later, at 79.88 years. By contrast, the age distribution for the upper extremity is unimodal, reaching its peak at 54.72 years for the "upper extremity" (Figure 2).

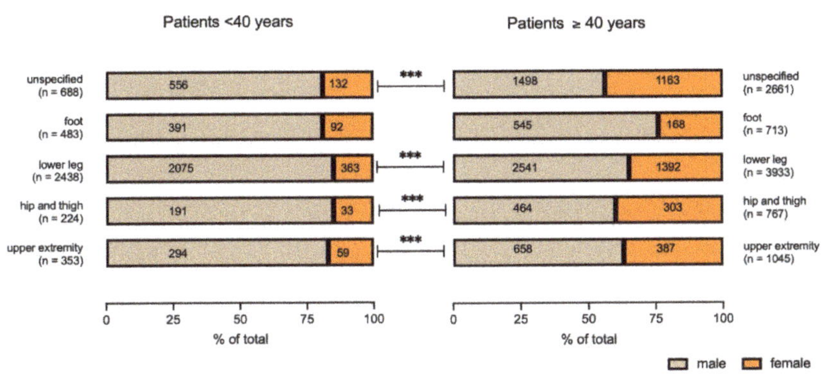

(A) **(B)**

Figure 1. Number and % of total of compartment syndromes categorized by localization (foot, upper extremity, hip and thigh, lower leg, or unspecified location) and age of patients ((**A**): <40 years; (**B**): ≥40 years). χ^2-test; *** $p < 0.001$.

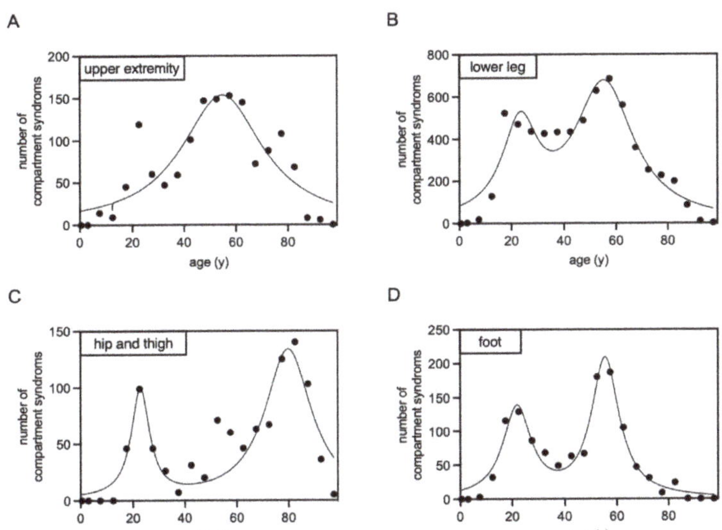

Figure 2. Non-linear regression analysis, employing Lorentzian distributions, was conducted on compartment syndrome cases following osteosynthesis between 2015 and 2022, categorized by the affected area ((**A**): upper extremity; (**B**): lower leg; (**C**): hip and thigh; (**D**): foot). The resulting graphs display the frequency of compartment syndromes in correlation with the patients' ages.

Throughout the analyzed period, all traumatic compartment syndromes exhibited a significant decline in cases per year, amounting to a reduction of 43.87 cases annually (Figure 3). A classification based on the sex also shows a significant decline of 36.04 cases per year for males and a not significant decline of 7.83 cases per year for females (Figure 3). Upon further classification based on localization, distinct patterns emerged. For the localizations "foot" and "lower leg", a statistically significant decrease in cases per year was identified ("foot": 16.67 fewer cases per year; "lower leg": 32.87 fewer cases per year). For "upper extremity" and "hip and thigh", there was also a decline in cases per year observed, but it was statistically not significant ("upper extremity": 3.78 fewer cases per year; "hip and thigh": 2.10 fewer cases per year) (Figure 4).

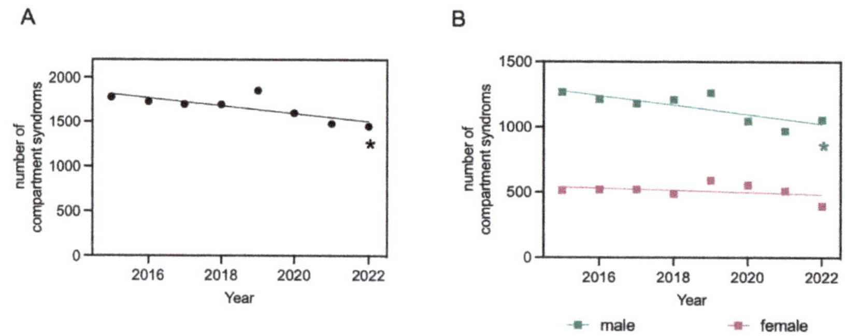

Figure 3. Compartment syndromes after osteosynthesis from 2015 to 2022. Linear regression function: y = −43.87x + 90,213; R^2 = 0.5842; * significantly non-zero slope of the line, evidenced by an F-statistic of 8.429 and a p-value of 0.03 (**A**). Compartment syndromes after osteosynthesis from 2015 to 2022, categorized by patients' sex (male and female). Linear regression function for males: y = −36.04x + 73,890; R^2 = 0.6325; * significantly non-zero slope of the line, evidenced by an F-statistic of 10.33 and p = 0.02. Linear regression function for females: y = −7.83x + 16,323; R^2 = 0.1147; slope of the line not significantly different from zero, evidenced by an F-statistic of 0.7774 and p = 0.41 (**B**).

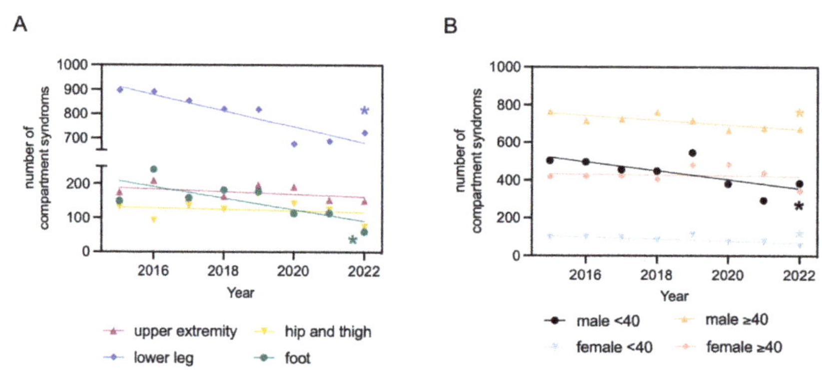

Figure 4. Compartment syndromes after osteosynthesis from 2015 to 2022, categorized by localization (foot, upper extremity, hip and thigh, lower leg). Linear regression function for the foot: y = −16.76x + 33,983; R^2 = 0.5652; * significantly non-zero slope of the line, evidenced by an F-statistic of 7.8 and p = 0.03. Linear regression function for the upper extremity: y = −3.786x + 7816; R^2 = 0.1794; slope of the line not significantly different from zero, evidenced by an F-statistic of 1.312 and p = 0.3. Linear regression function for the hip and thigh: y = −2.107x + 4377; R^2 = 0.03103; slope of the line not significantly different from zero, evidenced by an F-statistic of 0.1922 and p = 0.68. Linear regression function for the lower leg: y = −32.87x + 67,143; R^2 = 0.8277; * significantly non-zero slope of the line, evidenced by an F-statistic of 28.83 and p = 0.002 (**A**). Compartment syndromes after osteosynthesis from 2015 to 2022, categorized by patients age (<40 years and ≥40 years) and sex (male and female). Linear regression function for males under 40: y = −23.68x + 48,234; R^2 = 0.501; * significantly non-zero slope of the line, evidenced by an F-statistic of 6.025 and p = 0.05. Linear regression function for males over 40: y = −12.36x + 25,656; R^2 = 0.6429; * significantly non-zero slope of the line, evidenced by an F-statistic of 10.8 and p = 0.02. Linear regression function for females under 40: y = −5.750x + 11,691; R^2 = 0.5522; * significantly non-zero slope of the line, evidenced by an F-statistic of 7.398 and p = 0.03. Linear regression function for females over 40: y = −2.083x + 4632; R^2 = 0.01332; slope of the line not significantly different from zero, evidenced by an F-statistic of 0.08101 and p = 0.79 (**B**).

The subgroup analysis further confirms a yearly decrease in the incidence of compartment syndrome following osteosynthesis. Notably, a significant yearly decrease was observed in all male patient groups, with a reduction of 23.68 cases in males under 40 and 12.36 cases in males over 40. Among females under 40, the data also indicate a significant yearly decrease, with 5.75 fewer cases. However, for females over 40, the yearly reduction was not statistically significant, showing only a modest decrease of 2.08 cases (Figure 4).

4. Discussion

Our study uncovered clear trends and demographic features regarding compartment syndrome (CS) following trauma. Predominantly, cases were observed in the lower leg (44.4%), with a notable proportion occurring in the upper extremities (10.5%). These data are consistent with the literature. Notably, McQueen et al. demonstrated that fractures are the primary cause of CS at a rate of 69%, with the most prevalent location being the diaphysis of the tibia (36%), followed by the distal radius as the second most common site [15].

Our research examined 13,305 cases of traumatic compartment syndromes that were treated concurrently with osteosynthetic procedures, recorded in Germany from 2015 to 2022. Data from the German Statistical Office indicate that the country's average population during this period was approximately 83,053,327 [17]. This translates to an incidence rate of 2 per 100,000 individuals for traumatic compartment syndrome. With this incidence, the compartment syndrome following trauma represents a rare clinical entity that needs more attention.

A significant gender-based difference was observed, revealing a higher incidence of traumatic compartment syndromes in males compared to females, resulting in a female-to-male ratio of approximately 1:2.3 across all anatomical locations, including the upper extremity, thigh, lower leg, and foot. One plausible explanation for this observation is the greater likelihood of men being involved in high-energy accidents, often resulting in diverse bone fractures [18]. Additionally, McQueen et al. proposed that young men possess a larger proportion of muscle, while the fascial shell does not proportionally expand, potentially contributing to the observed patterns. Conversely, older men exhibit reduced muscular tissue, allowing more space for muscle swelling following injury [15]. Most studies indicate that youth is one of the strongest predictors for developing CS [19,20].

In our investigation, a bimodal pattern in the age distribution was observed for most anatomical locations, with initial peaks at 22 to 23 years, followed by a second peak at 55 years of age. Interestingly, the upper extremity displayed a unimodal pattern, peaking at 55 years. Despite indications in the dataset of a bimodal age distribution curve for the upper extremity group, its statistical significance was not confirmed across different statistical models. A plausible explanation for the prominence of the 55-year age group could be the occurrence of a midlife crisis, often experienced between ages 40 and 60. In this context, some individuals may engage in riskier activities or sports like motorcycling. Studies have shown that older victims of motorcycle crashes typically present with more severe injuries than their younger counterparts [21,22].

Furthermore, the period from 1955 to 1969 in Germany corresponds to the baby boomer generation [23]. Shoob et al. demonstrated that Baby Boomers significantly impacted the absolute numbers of hospitalizations for coronary heart disease and stroke in 2000 compared to individuals aged 45–54 in 1990 and 1980 [24]. This demographic phenomenon could contribute to an increased incidence of compartment syndrome within this specific age group. Interestingly, the second peak in the age distribution for "hip and thigh" was considerably later at 79.88 years. This could be explained by the increased incidence of femoral fractures in elderly patients combined with an oral anticoagulation therapy [25].

We observed a temporal declining trend in the incidence of compartment syndrome in our study, despite the increasing incidence of fractures in Germany from 2009 to 2019 [25]. The decline in traumatic compartment syndrome could be attributed to several factors. Advancements in surgical techniques and technologies, including osteosynthesis, have led to more precise and less invasive surgeries, potentially reducing the likelihood of complications like compartment syndrome. Enhanced imaging modalities, improved fixation devices, and better preoperative planning might collectively contribute to a decrease in postoperative complications.

Increased awareness among healthcare professionals about the risk factors and early signs of compartment syndrome could also play a crucial role in the observed decline of CS. Emphasis on medical education to monitor patients for symptoms of CS leads to earlier detection and intervention. As noted, the diagnosis of CS and the decision for surgical intervention remain challenging, evidenced by a study highlighting diverse rates of diagnosis and therapeutic interventions for CS [26]. Improving educational initiatives, raising awareness of CS, and focused sensitization may have resulted in a reduction in the indications for hasty or even unnecessary fasciotomies.

Recent diagnostic tools for identifying CS, such as continuous intracompartmental pressure monitoring, have demonstrated high sensitivity and specificity and should be considered for all high-risk patients [27]. This may contribute to further declining numbers. Moreover, the cautious approach to diagnosing compartment syndrome might also be a factor. Additionally, advances in rehabilitation strategies and postoperative care, focusing on minimizing swelling and optimizing tissue healing, may contribute to the reduction in the incidence of compartment syndromes. It is essential to consider these factors and their collective influence on the observed decline.

While many investigations have focused on individuals treated at a single trauma center, our study utilized a dataset from the Federal Statistical Office of Germany, covering 2015 to 2022. These data span diagnoses, treatments, and patient demographics, collected from numerous healthcare facilities across the nation. This comprehensive dataset allows for a thorough examination of demographic trends across Germany. Utilizing internationally recognized coding systems like the International Classification of Diseases (ICD) for diagnoses and the German procedure classification system (OPS) for treatments, the data maintain a high level of consistency. This standardization is crucial and allows a comparison with other datasets. However, the data source is not without its limitations. One of the primary concerns is the potential for coding errors and inconsistencies. Despite the standardization, data entry mistakes or variations in interpreting coding guidelines are possible. Additionally, since the data are tailored more for administrative and financial purposes, it often lacks detailed clinical information. In our dataset, approximately a quarter of cases lacked precise localization classification, highlighting one of our concerns. It is also possible that different hospitals and healthcare providers might employ varying practices in coding and data entry, which could introduce biases into the dataset. Additionally, our study included only traumatic compartment syndromes combined with simultaneously osteosynthetic treatment. Other traumatic causes such as spontaneous bleeding into a compartment, injection of pressurized fluid into the compartment, or a too-tight cast and all non-traumatic compartment syndromes were excluded [28,29]. Initially, we aimed to include all patients with traumatic compartment syndrome. Unfortunately, the billing data provided by the Statistical Office of Germany were not specific enough to answer this question, because non-traumatic compartment syndromes (e.g., after revascularization) were included in the dataset. To overcome this analysis bias, we had to refine our search query and search for the coded diagnosis of compartment syndrome in combination with any osteosynthesis that was performed during the same hospital stay. By doing so, we had the advantage of excluding non-traumatic compartment syndromes from our analysis but, on the other hand, faced the disadvantage of not being able to identify isolated traumatic compartment syndromes that did not require osteosynthesis. This approach made our results more accurate and specific to our research question.

Our current study provides a snapshot of compartment syndromes in Germany, offering insights within specific temporal and regional boundaries. The reasons behind the observed decrease in the number of compartment syndrome cases warrant further exploration in subsequent clinical studies. To this end, both prospective and retrospective clinical investigations are of great significance, as they can offer a deeper understanding of the underlying factors contributing to this trend.

Author Contributions: Conceptualization, P.H. and I.S.; methodology, A.E.; validation, F.H., D.R. and M.W.; formal analysis, I.S.; investigation, I.S., A.E. and P.H.; resources, M.R. and I.S.; data curation, T.H. and I.S.; writing—original draft preparation, P.H.; writing—review and editing, A.E., T.H., M.W., F.H., I.S. and M.W.; visualization, I.S.; supervision, M.R. All authors have read and agreed to the published version of the manuscript.

Funding: This publication was supported by the Open Access Publication Fund of the University of Wuerzburg.

Institutional Review Board Statement: Not applicable.

Informed Consent Statement: Not applicable.

Data Availability Statement: All source data can be downloaded from the URL https://github.com/ioannis-stratos/compartment (generated and accessed on 7 January 2024).

Conflicts of Interest: The authors declare no conflicts of interest.

References

1. Erdös, J.; Dlaska, C.; Szatmary, P.; Humenberger, M.; Vécsei, V.; Hajdu, S. Acute compartment syndrome in children: A case series in 24 patients and review of the literature. *Int. Orthop.* **2011**, *35*, 569–575. [CrossRef]
2. Mauser, N.; Gissel, H.; Henderson, C.; Hao, J.; Hak, D.; Mauffrey, C. Acute lower-leg compartment syndrome. *Orthopedics* **2013**, *36*, 619–624. [PubMed]
3. Shadgan, B.; Menon, M.; O'Brien, P.J.; Reid, W.D. Diagnostic techniques in acute compartment syndrome of the leg. *J. Orthop. Trauma* **2008**, *22*, 581–587. [CrossRef] [PubMed]
4. Smith, A.; Chitre, V.; Deo, H. Acute gluteal compartment syndrome: Superior gluteal artery rupture following a low energy injury. *BMJ Case Rep.* **2012**, *2012*, bcr2012007710. [CrossRef] [PubMed]
5. Davaine, J.M.; Lintz, F.; Cappelli, M.; Chaillou, P.; Gouin, F.; Patra, P.; Gouëffic, Y. Acute compartment syndrome of the thigh secondary to isolated common femoral vessel injury: An unusual etiology. *Ann. Vasc. Surg.* **2013**, *27*, 802.e1–4. [CrossRef] [PubMed]
6. Coban, Y.K. Rhabdomyolysis, compartment syndrome and thermal injury. *World J. Crit. Care Med.* **2014**, *3*, 1–7. [CrossRef] [PubMed]
7. Jones, G.; Thompson, K.; Johnson, M. Acute compartment syndrome after minor trauma in a patient with undiagnosed mild haemophilia B. *Lancet* **2013**, *382*, 1678. [CrossRef]
8. Kleshinski, J.; Bittar, S.; Wahlquist, M.; Ebraheim, N.; Duggan, J.M. Review of compartment syndrome due to group A streptococcal infection. *Am. J. Med. Sci.* **2008**, *336*, 265–269. [CrossRef]
9. Defraigne, J.O.; Pincemail, J. Local and systemic consequences of severe ischemia and reperfusion of the skeletal muscle. Physiopathology and prevention. *Acta Chir. Belg.* **1998**, *98*, 176–186. [CrossRef]
10. Chim, H.; Soltanian, H. Spontaneous compartment syndrome of the forearm in association with nephrotic syndrome and transient bacteremia. *J. Surg. Case Rep.* **2012**, *2012*, 11. [CrossRef] [PubMed]
11. Matsen, F.A., 3rd. A practical approach to compartmental syndromes. Part I. Definition, theory, and pathogenesis. *Instr. Course Lect.* **1983**, *32*, 88–92. [PubMed]
12. Sheridan, G.W.; Matsen, F.A., 3rd. Fasciotomy in the treatment of the acute compartment syndrome. *J. Bone Jt. Surg. Am.* **1976**, *58*, 112–115. [CrossRef]
13. von Keudell, A.G.; Weaver, M.J.; Appleton, P.T.; Bae, D.S.; Dyer, G.S.M.; Heng, M.; Jupiter, J.B.; Vrahas, M.S. Diagnosis and treatment of acute extremity compartment syndrome. *Lancet* **2015**, *386*, 1299–1310. [CrossRef] [PubMed]
14. Donaldson, J.; Haddad, B.; Khan, W.S. The pathophysiology, diagnosis and current management of acute compartment syndrome. *Open Orthop. J.* **2014**, *8*, 185–193. [CrossRef]
15. McQueen, M.M.; Gaston, P.; Court-Brown, C.M. Acute compartment syndrome. Who is at risk? *J. Bone Jt. Surg. Br.* **2000**, *82*, 200–203. [CrossRef]
16. Lollo, L.; Grabinsky, A. Clinical and functional outcomes of acute lower extremity compartment syndrome at a Major Trauma Hospital. *Int. J. Crit. Illn. Inj. Sci.* **2016**, *6*, 133–142. [CrossRef]
17. Destatis. Available online: https://www.destatis.de/DE/Themen/Gesellschaft-Umwelt/Bevoelkerung/Bevoelkerungsstand/Tabellen/deutsche-nichtdeutsche-bevoelkerung-nach-geschlecht-deutschland.html (accessed on 20 June 2023).
18. Almigdad, A.; Mustafa, A.; Alazaydeh, S.; Alshawish, M.; Bani Mustafa, M.; Alfukaha, H. Bone Fracture Patterns and Distributions according to Trauma Energy. *Adv. Orthop.* **2022**, *2022*, 8695916. [CrossRef] [PubMed]
19. McQueen, M.M.; Duckworth, A.D.; Aitken, S.A.; Sharma, R.A.; Court-Brown, C.M. Predictors of Compartment Syndrome After Tibial Fracture. *J. Orthop. Trauma* **2015**, *29*, 451–455. [CrossRef]
20. Gamulin, A.; Wuarin, L.; Zingg, M.; Belinga, P.; Cunningham, G.; Gonzalez, A.I. Association between open tibia fractures and acute compartment syndrome: A retrospective cohort study. *Orthop. Traumatol. Surg. Res.* **2022**, *108*, 103188. [CrossRef]

21. Dischinger, P.C.; Ryb, G.E.; Ho, S.M.; Braver, E.R. Injury patterns and severity among hospitalized motorcyclists: A comparison of younger and older riders. *Annu. Proc. Assoc. Adv. Automot. Med.* **2006**, *50*, 237–249.
22. Dischinger, P.C.; Ryb, G.E.; Ho, S.M.; Burch, C.A. The association between age, injury, and survival to hospital among a cohort of injured motorcyclists. *Annu. Proc. Assoc. Adv. Automot. Med.* **2007**, *51*, 97–110.
23. Toczek, L.; Bosma, H.; Peter, R. Early retirement intentions: The impact of employment biographies, work stress and health among a baby-boomer generation. *Eur. J. Ageing* **2022**, *19*, 1479–1491. [CrossRef]
24. Shoob, H.D.; Croft, J.B.; Labarthe, D.R. Impact of Baby Boomers on hospitalizations for coronary heart disease and stroke in the United States. *Prev. Med.* **2007**, *44*, 447–451. [CrossRef]
25. Rupp, M.; Walter, N.; Pfeifer, C.; Lang, S.; Kerschbaum, M.; Krutsch, W.; Baumann, F.; Alt, V. The Incidence of Fractures Among the Adult Population of Germany–an Analysis From 2009 through 2019. *Dtsch. Arztebl. Int.* **2021**, *118*, 665–669.
26. O'Toole, R.V.; Whitney, A.; Merchant, N.; Hui, E.; Higgins, J.; Kim, T.T.; Sagebien, C. Variation in diagnosis of compartment syndrome by surgeons treating tibial shaft fractures. *J. Trauma.* **2009**, *67*, 735–741. [CrossRef]
27. McQueen, M.M.; Duckworth, A.D.; Aitken, S.A.; Court-Brown, C.M. The estimated sensitivity and specificity of compartment pressure monitoring for acute compartment syndrome. *J. Bone Jt. Surg. Am.* **2013**, *95*, 673–677. [CrossRef] [PubMed]
28. Dumontier, C.; Sautet, A.; Man, M.; Bennani, M.; Apoil, A. Entrapment and compartment syndromes of the upper limb in haemophilia. *J. Hand Surg. Br.* **1994**, *19*, 427–429. [CrossRef] [PubMed]
29. Seiler, J.G., 3rd; Valadie, A.L., 3rd; Drvaric, D.M.; Frederick, R.W.; Whitesides, T.E., Jr. Perioperative compartment syndrome. A report of four cases. *J. Bone Jt. Surg. Am.* **1996**, *78*, 600–602. [CrossRef] [PubMed]

Journal of
Clinical Medicine

MDPI

Review

A Novel Surgical Treatment Management Algorithm for Elbow Posterolateral Rotatory Instability (PLRI) Based on the Common Extensor Origin Integrity

Christos Koukos [1,2], Michail Kotsapas [3], Konstantinos Sidiropoulos [4,5,*], Aurélien Traverso [6,7], Kerem Bilsel [8,9], Fredy Montoya [10] and Paolo Arrigoni [7]

1 Medical Center Wuppertal, 42329 Wuppertal, Germany; koukos_christos@hotmail.com
2 Sports Trauma and Pain Institute, 54655 Thessaloniki, Greece
3 Orthopaedic Department, General Hospital of Naousa, 59200 Naousa, Greece
4 Medical School of Patras, University of Patras, 26504 Patras, Greece
5 Emergency Department, Papageorgiou General Hospital of Thessaloniki, 54635 Thessaloniki, Greece
6 Orthopaedic Department, Centre Hospitalier Universitaire Vaudois (CHUV), 1011 Lausanne, Switzerland
7 ASST Pini-CTO, 20122 Milan, Italy
8 Faculty of Medicine, Acibadem Mehmet Ali Aydınlar University, 34752 Instanbul, Turkey; kerem.bilsel@acibadem.com
9 Orthopaedics and Traumatology Department, FulyaAcibadem Hospital, 34349 Instanbul, Turkey
10 Sanatorio Aleman Clinic, Universidad de Concepcion, Concepcion 4070386, Chile; fmontoya@puc.cl
* Correspondence: kcdroq@yahoo.gr; Tel.: +30-2313323408

Abstract: Background: Here, we introduce a comprehensive treatment algorithm for posterolateral rotatory instability (PLRI) of the elbow, a condition affecting elbow mobility. We outline a diagnostic approach and a novel surgical management plan through the arthroscopic surgeon's point of view. **Methods**: The central focus of this management approach is the integrity of common extensor origin (CEO). High clinical suspicion must be evident to diagnose PLRI. Special clinical and imaging tests can confirm PLRI but sometimes the final confirmation is established during the arthroscopic treatment. The most appropriate treatment is determined by the degree of CEO integrity. **Results**: The treatment strategy varies with the CEO's condition: intact or minor tears require arthroscopic lateral collateral ligament imbrication, while extensive tears may need plication reinforced with imbrication or, in cases of retraction, a triceps tendon autograft reconstruction of the lateral ulnar collateral ligament alongside CEO repair. These approaches aim to manage residual instability and are complemented using a tailored rehabilitation protocol to optimize functional outcomes. **Conclusion**: PLRI is a unique clinical condition and should be treated likewise. This algorithm offers valuable insights for diagnosing and treating PLRI, enhancing therapeutic decision-making.

Keywords: posterolateral rotational instability (PLRI) of elbow; PLRI diagnosis; clinical tests for elbow instability; common extensors origin (CEO) integrity; PLRI surgical treatment algorithm

1. Introduction

The elbow is a congruent joint presenting inherent stability due to bone morphology (ulnohumeral joint) and anatomic restraints, both static and dynamic. The ulnohumeral joint serves as a primary static stabilizer, with the medial collateral ligament (MCL) and the lateral collateral ligament complex (LCLC) as the major stabilizing ligaments [1,2]. Instability arises from the insufficiency of these structures due to trauma or degeneration. A significant lesion that leads to the posterolateral rotatory instability (PLRI) of the elbow is a dysfunction of the ulnar component of the lateral collateral ligamentous complex (LUCL) [3–6]. PLRI was first described by O'Driscoll et al. [7,8], and is the most common form of chronic elbow instability. This entity is characterized by a wide range of clinical manifestations, ranging from minor laxity to gross instability and elbow dislocations [3,9].

Consequently, addressing PLRI is challenging and entails a thorough physical examination, adequate imaging, and meticulous preoperative planning. Even though the importance of the common extensor origin (CEO) as a secondary lateral static stabilizer has been highlighted in the literature [10], to our knowledge, there is a lack of clarity on whether its condition should be taken into consideration systematically. This review strives to elucidate the pathophysiology leading to PLRI and to suggest a PLRI management algorithm that takes CEO integrity into account.

2. Anatomy and Considerations

The condition known as posterolateral rotatory instability (PLRI) was described by O'Driscoll et al. in 1991 as an instability pattern of the elbow that results from an weakened lateral ulnar collateral ligament (LUCL), which is a restraint to varus stress and acts to stabilize the radial head from posterior subluxation or dislocation [8]. Recent studies suggest the potential for broader compromise within the lateral collateral ligamentous complex [11,12]. Its etiology is mainly a consequence of trauma in 94% of patients, involving either an elbow dislocation or a fall with outstretched and supinated forearm [7,13,14]. A common mechanism is a fall onto an outstretched hand, leading to axial loading and elbow supination [4,15–19]. Minor repetitive microtrauma during sports or everyday activities also applies a substantial amount of stress on the LUCL, and if not addressed adequately results in the ligament's attenuation and dysfunction, and ultimately PLRI [2]. Iatrogenic lesions, often a surgical complication, can also occur after multiple steroid injections during treatment for persistent lateral epicondylitis [2,15,20]. Excessive stripping of the lateral condyle during the open approach, aggressive arthroscopic or open approaches for the common extensor origin (CEO), or capsular release pose a risk of compromising the LCLC's function due to its close anatomic proximity [2,10,15]. Repeated steroid injections affect the quality of both the CEO and the lateral stabilizers, leading consequently to CEO weakening and deficiency [10,19]. To summarize, it can be either an iatrogenic complication of continuous corticosteroid injections or of lateral epicondylitis surgery, as well as from cubitus varus injury due to the attenuation of ligaments.

Schnetzke M et al. [21] support that all simple elbow dislocations result in LCLC injuries, while magnetic resonance imaging (MRI) signal abnormalities in the CEO are evident in 39% of patients. Kim YS et al. [22] found that all patients with lateral epicondylitis present various degrees of CEO lesions and an LCLC dysfunction is present in 55%. They concluded that as the grade of the CEO lesion increases, so too does the incidence of potential PLRI in patients with lateral epicondylitis. The size of the CEO tear, the grade of CEO abnormality, and the presence of extensor muscle edema are the key factors related to the surgical management of lateral epicondylitis [23]. These data suggest a mutual relationship between CEO condition and LCLC integrity, both anatomically and functionally.

According to O'Driscoll, when the LUCL is not functional, the radial head rolls off the capitellum during forearm supination and subluxates posterolaterally. The ulnohumeral joint begins to gap and, as the pattern of instability continues, the entire elbow joint may dislocate. When the radial collateral ligament (RCL) does not heal properly and is nonfunctional, the radial head rolls off of the capitellum during forearm supination. As the radial head subluxates posterolaterally, the ulnohumeral joint begins to gap and, as the pattern of instability continues, the entire elbow joint may dislocate [8]. This concept has been debated recently throughout the literature demonstrating not a single dysfunctional lateral elbow anatomical structure but many of them, including radial collateral ligament, annular ligament (partially), and/or the common extensor mechanism [24]. Dunning et al. stated that to achieve PLRI, both the LUCL and the RCL must be sectioned. It has also been demonstrated that sectioning the anterior band of the lateral collateral complex induces instability, suggesting that an intact LUCL alone cannot stabilize the elbow [11,25]. Therefore, PLRI is not merely the result of an elbow dislocation but rather a range of injuries.

3. Clinical Presentation and Diagnosis

PLRI may have various clinical presentations with insidious courses of symptoms, making its diagnosis challenging to the inexperienced physician. Patients often complain of discomfort or lateral-sided pain during activities that require extension and supination, often associated with locking or catching during extension of the elbow at 40° flexion [8,24]. Most patients with chronic PLRI may have a normal appearance of the elbow with a full range of motion, and palpation may not trigger any pain [26].

Patients with chronic or subtle instability can be easily examined and assessed through clinical examinations such as the pivot shift test, the posterior radiocapitellar test, and the push-up and chair-rise tests [27]. It is crucial to note that the sensitivity of these tests heavily relies on the clinician's experience and the patient's tolerance [28]. Microinstability can be easily overlooked [9].

Plain X-rays are a necessity in the setting of acute elbow trauma to evaluate articular congruency and osseous injuries, while more complex cases may require investigation with Computed Tomography (CT) to reveal occult fractures or support preoperative planning [28]. Ultrasound (US) requires user experience and allows for real-time dynamic elbow examination [29,30]. Moreover, it is a very useful and inexpensive diagnostic tool to evaluate soft tissue integrity, particularly in lateral epicondylitis, with a reported sensitivity of 80% and a specificity of 50% [31]. According to a cadaveric study, US is superior to MRI in recognizing LUCL, demonstrating higher sensitivity and accuracy [6]. Nonetheless, MRI remains the modality of choice in soft tissue investigation [28]. Apart from ligament tears, scar tissue, or CEO ruptures, additional joint lesions, such as chondral lesions or osseous oedema, can also be evaluated with MRI [16,28]. Tendinous and ligamentous lesions are best evaluated in T2-weighted images [22,31,32]. In MRI, a radiocapitellar incongruity of more than 3.4 mm has an absolute positive predictive value for a pathology affecting elbow stability, while an incongruity of less than 0.3 mm has an absolute negative predictive value. In addition, a ulnohumeral incongruity of more than 1.5 mm has an absolute positive predictive value and less than 0.3 mm has a negative predictive value, excluding elbow instability, according to Hackl et al. [28]. A coexisting CEO injury correlates with increased incongruency on MRI [28]. Fluoroscopy under local anesthesia may show the radial head and proximal ulna posterolaterally subluxated and rotated [33].

The proximity of the LCLC and the CEO highlights the necessity of carefully evaluating the integrity of each structure if the other one is compromised. Bredella et al. advocate that lateral epicondylitis often co-occurs with LUCL lesions [32]. Furthermore, an acute traumatic LUCL rupture may be accompanied by a CEO rupture or avulsion [31,34]. According to Walz et al., CEO lesions in lateral epicondylitis are categorized as mild, moderate, and severe [31]. Mild lateral epicondylitis corresponds to CEO tendinosis or minor partial tears affecting less than 20% of the tendon thickness. Moderate lateral epicondylitis involves intermediate tears affecting more than 20% but less than 80% of the tendon thickness. Severe lateral epicondylitis is indicated by a high-grade partial-thickness tear (more than 80% of tendon thickness) or a full-thickness CEO tear [23,31,32].

4. Unique Features

Baker's arthroscopic classification of CEO lesions was groundbreaking when it was published, but it has limited predictive value for patient outcomes [35]. We find an MRI-based, preoperative algorithm for classifying CEO integrity more beneficial as it determines the therapeutic course of action before the surgery, as opposed to during it. Treatment algorithms for acute and chronic elbow instability have been offered by Savoie [36] and van Riet [37], but they do not consider CEO integrity. O'Driscoll et al. [10] argue that if the CEO deficiency exceeds an undetermined limit, LCLC reconstruction may be subjected to high strain and a higher failure rate. We propose a treatment algorithm that addresses this issue, considering CEO quality without quantifying a threshold. The ideal approach for an arthroscopic surgeon is to formulate a preoperative plan using objective data from an MRI and confirm the diagnosis via arthroscopic assessment. These features are lacking in currently available protocols. A practical and straightforward management protocol is needed. Due to these limitations, we have developed and implemented a new treatment algorithm that emphasizes clinical features and only employs an open technique when absolutely necessary.

In summary, we aim to propose a PLRI treatment protocol that achieves the following:

1. It is straightforward to grasp.
2. It directly applies to clinical settings without requiring complex procedures.
3. It utilizes arthroscopic minimally invasive techniques, which minimize potential iatrogenic instability; in contrast, open procedures can exacerbate elbow instability, which is challenging to rectify [38].
4. It is contingent on the integrity of the CEO, whether it is intact, has a moderate or extensive partial tear, or is completely ruptured with or without retraction. This evaluation can be conveniently conducted via MRI.

PLRI is categorized into three stages. Stage 1 is characterized by the posterolateral rotatory subluxation of the elbow, which a pivot-shift test can confirm. Stage 2 involves an incomplete dislocation of the elbow, with the coronoid process positioned under the trochlea. In Stage 3, a full elbow dislocation occurs, moving the coronoid process behind the humerus. There are also three subcategories for Stage 3: 3A, where the MCL anterior band remains intact, allowing the elbow to remain stable against valgus stress post reduction; 3B, where the anterior band of the MCL is disrupted, leading to elbow instability under valgus stress post reduction; and 3C, where complete elbow instability is caused by the stripping of all the humerus' soft tissues [8].

5. PLRI Treatment

MRI evaluation of CEO integrity is significant for the development of this proposed algorithm. Effective preoperative planning contributes to improved postoperative results. This treatment pathway can be determined after stress examination during arthroscopy [36], and postintervention arthroscopic instability evaluation can be repeated and compared to the preintervention examination.

While the Walz classification of CEO condition is useful, it has proven challenging to integrate directly into a treatment protocol, as it is designed specifically for diagnosing lateral epicondylitis. As such, we suggest a new integrity classification for the CEO that can better guide our PLRI treatment plan (Figure 1). First, PLRI must be confirmed; if not, we conduct an elbow arthroscopy for diagnosis. When the CEO is either intact or has a moderate partial tear, we propose arthroscopic LCL imbrication as the preferred treatment (Figures 2–6). If there is extensive partial CEO rupture or complete rupture without retraction, arthroscopic LCL plication may yield good or excellent results. In cases where the CEO is ruptured and retracted, we recommend reconstructing the LUCL with a triceps tendon autograft and repairing the CEO through an open procedure.

Arrigoni et al. [9] evaluated pathologic lateral ligamentous laxity with the presence of three arthroscopic signs: the annular-drive through sign, the loose collar sign, and the pull-up sign of R-LCL (radial component of the lateral collateral ligament). In addition, any coexisting intra-articular pathology can be evaluated and addressed. Patients suffering from subtle instability may have an intact CEO or a moderate partial CEO tear on MRI. These patients may be managed with a minimally invasive soft tissue procedure, such as LCL imbrication [17]. This procedure offers a sufficient alternative option compared to open reconstruction surgery, with equivalent postoperative stability rates [3,17], and aims to regain tension of the lateral stabilizers, such as the LCLC, the lateral capsule, and the anconeus muscle [3]. The patient is first placed in the lateral decubitus position under sedation and regional anesthesia. Range of motion is documented with mobility maneuvers. Stability is evaluated using varus and valgus stress tests, pivot-shift, and posterior drawer maneuvers. A hemostatic cuff is placed on the proximal third of the arm and insufflated. A mark is placed at the center of the lateral epicondyle as well as one indicating the direction of the LUCL. The elbow is insufflated with saline solution.

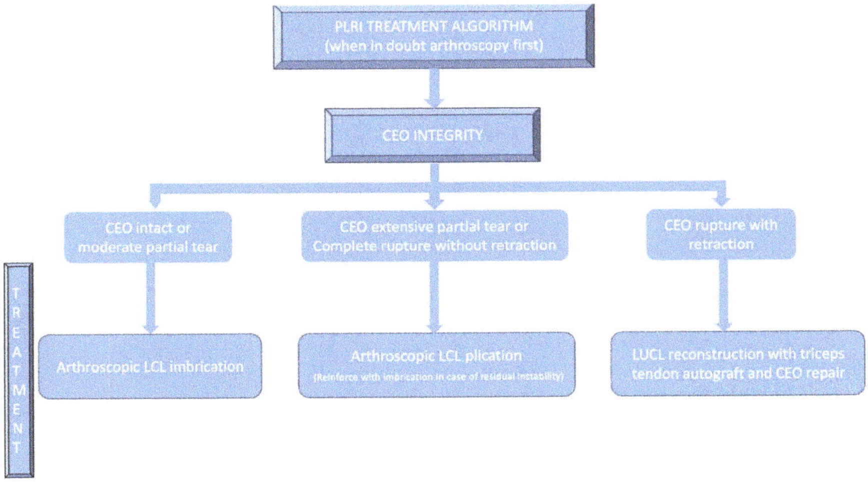

Figure 1. PLRI treatment algorithm according to CEO integrity.

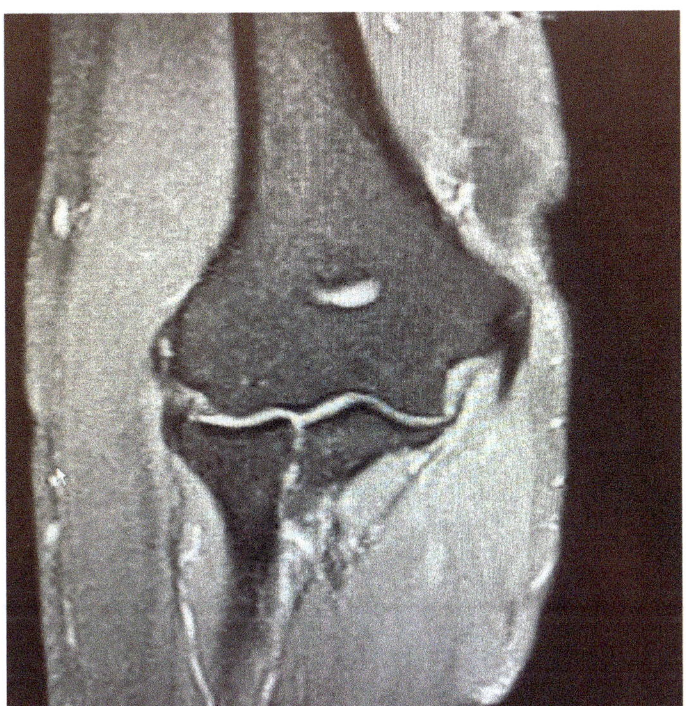

Figure 2. Minor partial CEO tear [courtesy of C.K.].

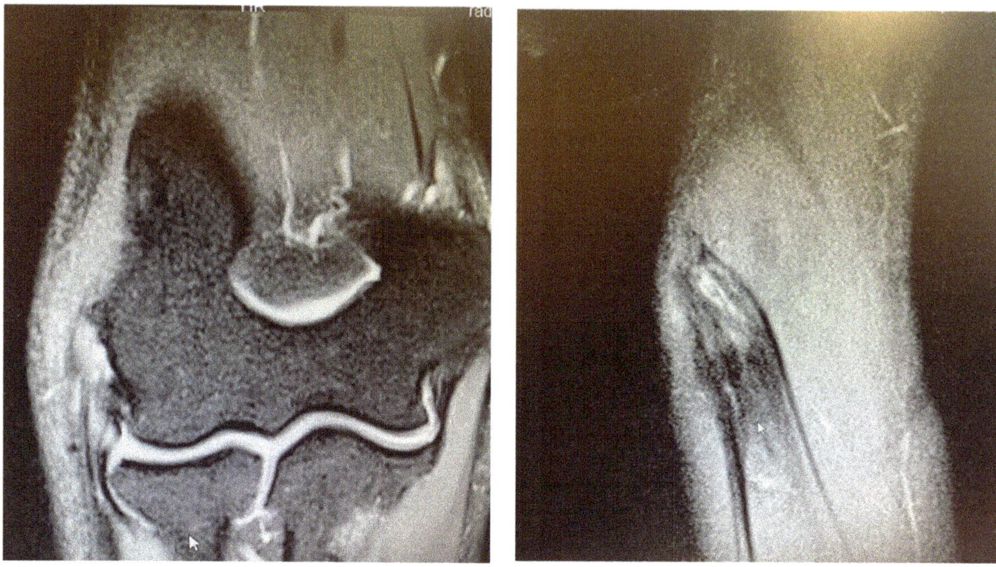

Figure 3. Extensive partial CEO tear [courtesy of C.K.].

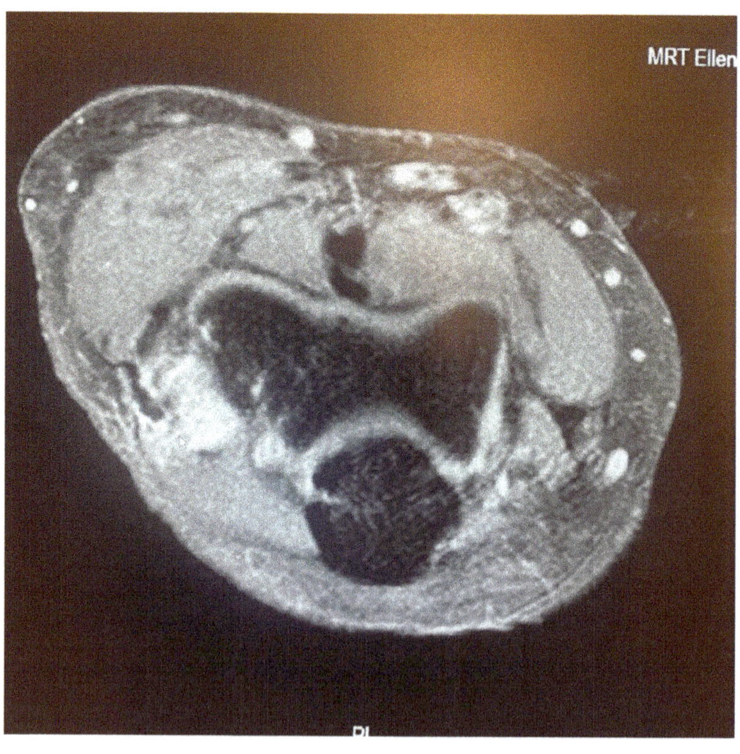

Figure 4. Complete CEO rupture [courtesy of C.K.].

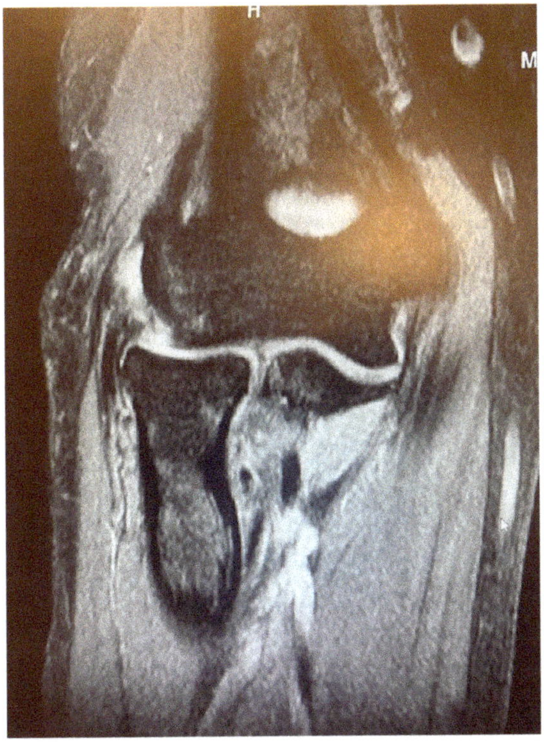

Figure 5. Complete CEO rupture without retraction [courtesy of C.K.].

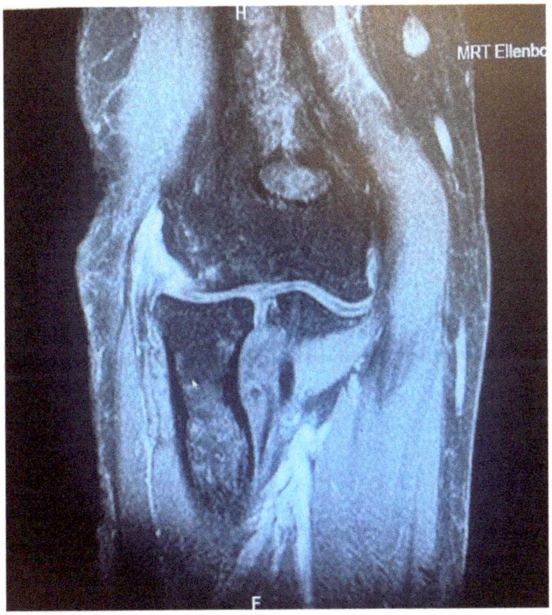

Figure 6. Complete CEO rupture with retraction and poor tendon quality [courtesy of C.K.].

The anterior compartment of the joint is visualized through an anteromedial portal. This allows us to demonstrate the opening of the radiohumeral joint by placing a feeler between the capitellum and the radial head. A high posterolateral portal is placed at the lateral tip of the olecranon to be able to visualize the posterior compartment, including the tip of the olecranon and the fossa (if any pathology is evident, a central posterior portal can be made to resolve said pathology). Valgus stress is applied to assess the integrity of the MCL under direct vision. In case the joint does not open, the MCL would be unharmed. Subsequently, the humerus–radial joint is visualized. The scope is pushed into the lateral gutter while a soft-spot portal is created to remove any synovium blocking the view. The arthroscopic rotatory instability test, the drive-through sign, and the trocar test, performed from the posterior compartment, help validate the diagnosis of PLRI [17]. Hypersupination with varus stress on the forearm will show the radial head subluxating posteriorly on the capitellum and the radiocapitellar joint line widening, while longitudinal pressure on the forearm may reveal more radiohumeral joint space gapping, the so-called pull test. An indirect indicator of lateral laxity is also the occasional sagging of the annular ligament [17].

A PDS II suture is threaded from the center of the epicondyle towards the radiohumeral joint using a suture passer (CHIA perc-passer, DePuy Synthes, Warsaw, IN, USA) and pulled out through the direct lateral portal with forceps. Another identical suture is directed towards the insertion of the LUCL in the radiohumeral joint from the subcutaneous edge of the ulna and retrieved via the same portal. This leaves two strands of PDS II sutures. The first enters the skin at the lateral epicondyle's center, moves through the capsule and LCL complex, and exits through the direct lateral portal. The second does the same, starting at the ulna's subcutaneous edge just below the LUCL insertion and passing through the anconeus, capsule, and LUCL. Both suture ends that exit through the direct lateral portal are tied together, forming a single suture line stretching from the lateral epicondyle to the ulna's subcutaneous edge. Finally, the four suture ends are drawn out through the direct lateral portal.

The test for rotational stability is conducted once more, in which the forearm is fully supinated, and a forced varus is performed with both loose and tight sutures. After tightening the sutures, the rotatory instability test results turn negative, indicating that the sutures can be tied together. After the scope is removed, each suture is tied separately, and the knots are concealed. The portals are then closed, and a posterior splint is placed on the elbow. Patients are then fitted with a hinged brace. Postoperative radiographs or radioscopy are performed to ensure that the joint remains in reduction. After the initial postoperative visit, the elbow may be placed in a hinged elbow brace to allow for gradual movement (within a range of 30–120° for 4 weeks). Exercises for the peri-scapular region, wrist, and hand are permitted. Immediate physical therapy is mandatory.

Patients with extensive partial or complete CEO ruptures, as evidenced by MRI scans, often see more benefits from an arthroscopic LCLC plication. This procedure, outlined by Savoie et al. [33], involves placing a double-loaded anchor at the isometric point on the capitellum's lateral side. Then, sutures are placed into the posterolateral gutter from the radial border of the ulna, moving distally to the proximal. The first of these sutures is delivered through the annular ligament into the joint. Using a portal, the sutures are collected subcutaneously and tensioned and knotted as the arthroscope is removed from the lateral gutter. If any residual instability is noticed during arthroscopy post intervention, the plicated lateral soft tissues can be augmented with imbrication. After the procedure, the patient is fitted with a hinged brace for 4 weeks, allowing for neutral forearm rotation and an elbow extension range of 30–120°. Strengthening exercises are generally started after the sixth week post operation and continue until the third month. To allow for adequate healing, full weight-bearing activities should be avoided for 3 months post operation (Figures 7–12).

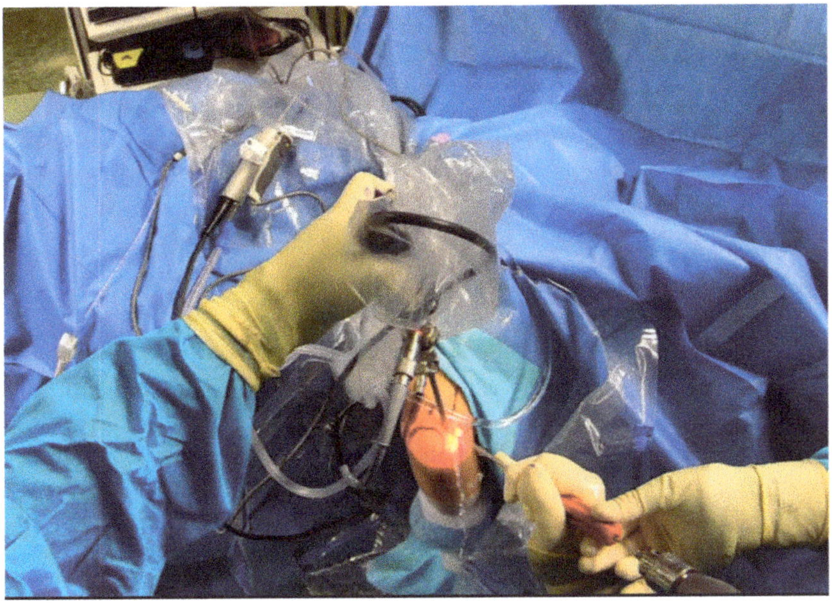

Figure 7. Arthroscopy. Drilling prior to anchor placement [courtesy of C.K.].

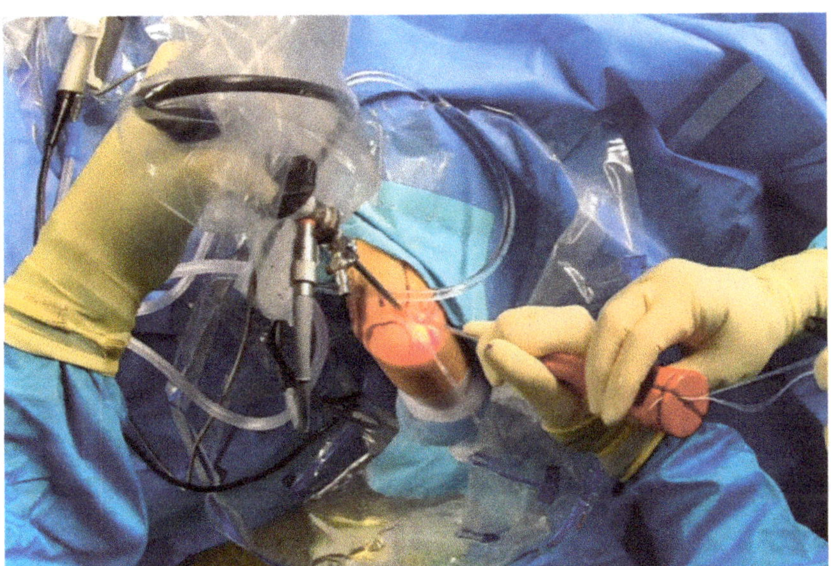

Figure 8. Anchor placement [courtesy of C.K.].

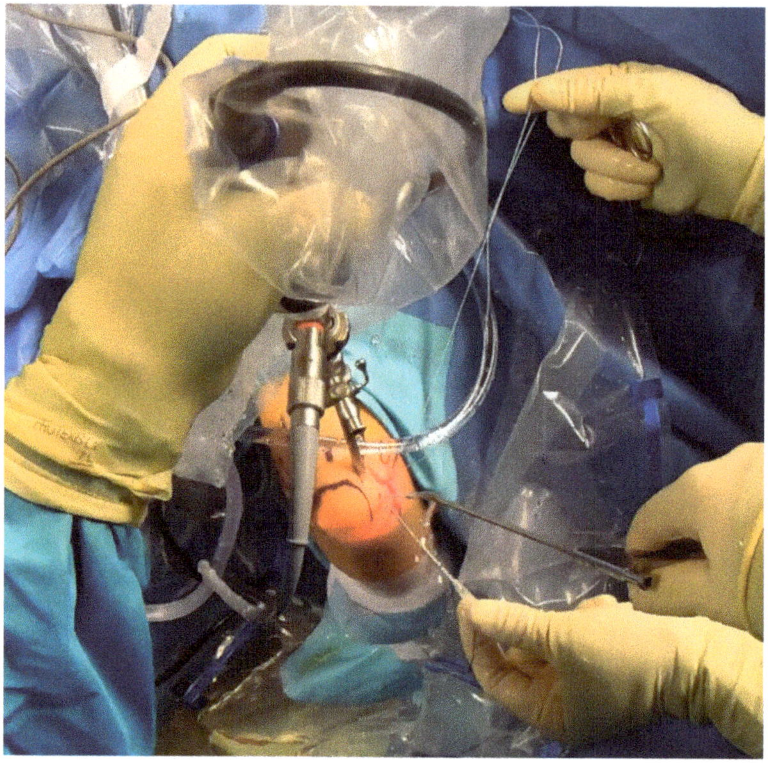

Figure 9. Suture shuttling by using a 14G needle [courtesy of C.K.].

Patients with a fully ruptured CEO and distal CEO retraction typically experience significant symptomatic instability. They need LUCL reconstruction with an autograft plus lateral epicondyle extensor repair [39]. Confirming PLRI via diagnostic arthroscopy should precede these procedures. Surgeons should carry out these interventions using an open procedure. As Dehlinger et al. outlined [40], the second step involves harvesting an ipsilateral triceps tendon autograft. This graft should measure at least 7 cm by 4.5 mm. The surgical technique from the primary author (C.K.) includes orienting the prepared graft with its ulnar side through a single cortical hole. This location should be at the annular ligament's intersection with the radial head and neck, facing the distal ulnar direction to match the LUCL's force vector. The graft's humeral end is inserted at the humeral isometry point through a 2 cm deep hole made in the proximal–dorsal direction. The graft's final ulnar position is secured with an anchor suture that also functions like a screw. The remaining suture then reinforces the fixation. On the humeral side, the graft's position is secured with FiberWire® (Arthrex, Naples, FL, USA), leaving a 2 cm intraosseous portion. Afterward, a tug on the graft secures it further with another suture anchor similar to a screw. Optimizing the humeral isometry point is next, following functional testing. The knotted FiberWire® threads should be threaded into the screw for added support. The CEO is then reattached to the lateral epicondyle using anchor sutures. For large defects, surgeons can insert a suture anchor into the lateral condyle's flexion side. After surgery, the patient wears a hinged brace set to allow extension/flexion from 30° to 120°. This continues for 4 weeks, followed by an additional 2 weeks without restrictions. The postoperative rehabilitation protocol includes extensor isometric exercises from the fourth week, followed by gradual weight training.

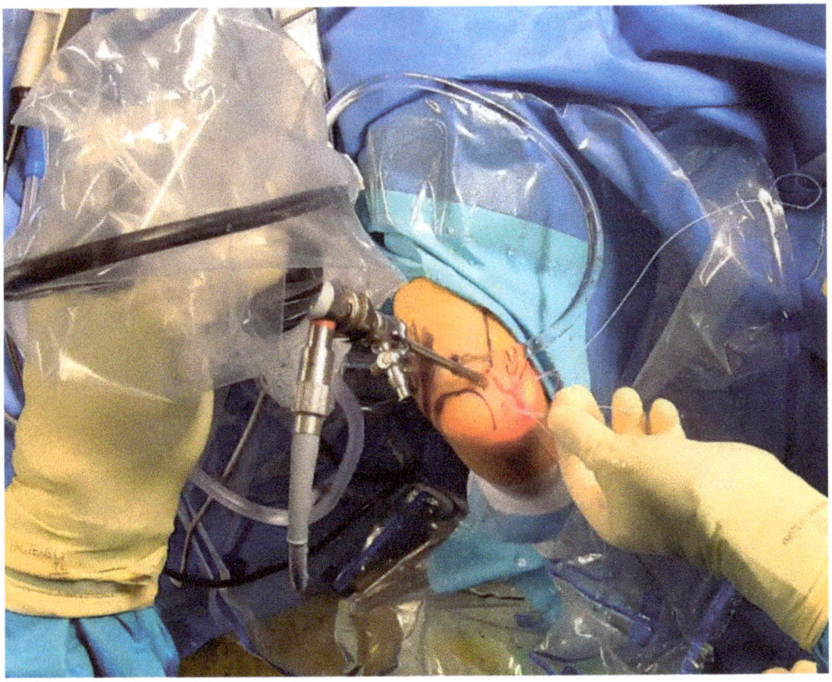

Figure 10. Suture shuttling (2nd stage) [courtesy of C.K.].

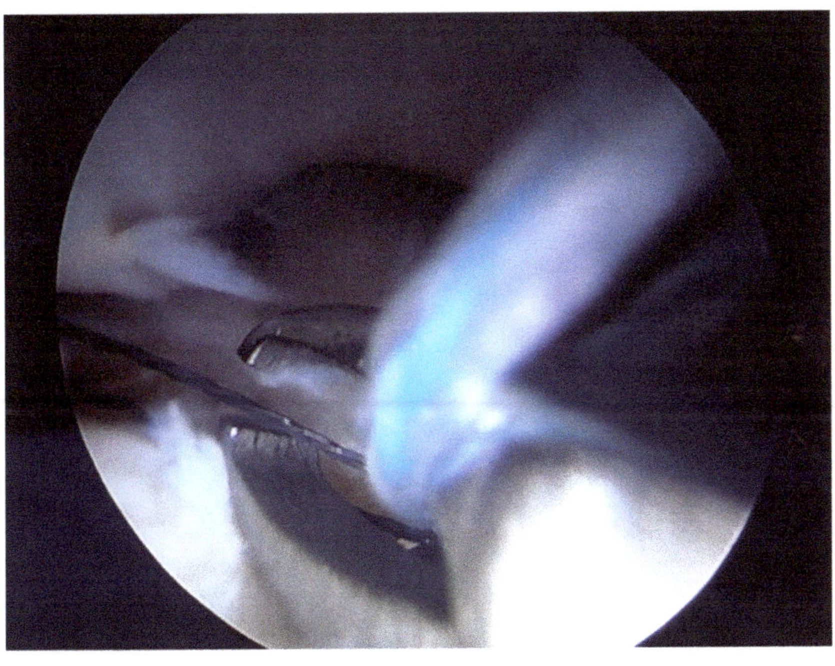

Figure 11. Arthroscopic view of suture shuttling [courtesy of C.K.].

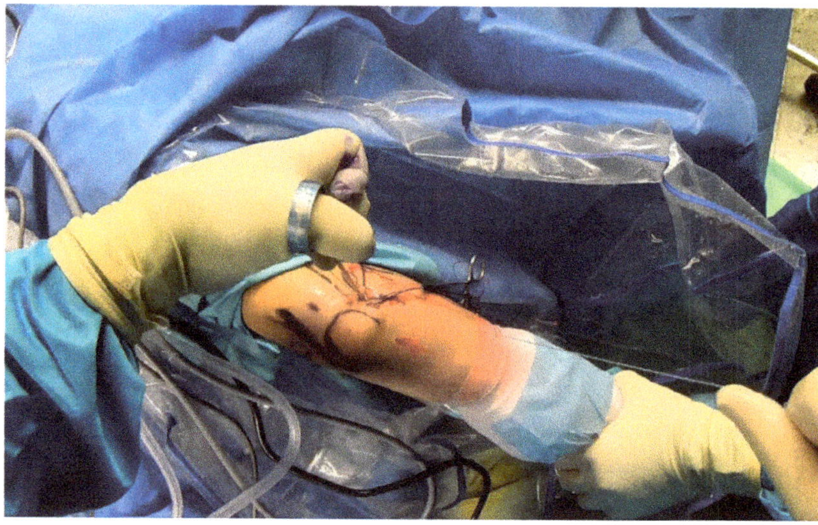

Figure 12. Final plication—suture tying by using sliding knots [courtesy of C.K.].

6. Discussion

Lateral elbow pain may be attributed to bony structure lesions (humerus, radius, and ulna), ligament lesions (LCLC), tendons (CEO), and nerves (branches of the radial nerve), making diagnostic and therapeutic management demanding [41,42]. PLRI and lateral epicondylitis may coexist, especially if lateral epicondylitis is persistent, misguiding the examiner [19,36]. As described by Arrigoni et al. [9], Symptomatic Minor Instability of the Lateral Elbow (SMILE) is a recently introduced clinical condition characterized by lateral ligamentous laxity usually associated with at least one intra-articular lesion, which can also mimic or accompany persistent lateral epicondylitis. Repeated corticosteroid injections or lateral elbow surgery for addressing lateral epicondylitis may raise clinical suspicion of lateral stabilizers' compromise and potential PLRI in cases of persistent pain [20,34]. A thorough clinical and imaging investigation is required to avoid misdiagnosis. Since O'Driscoll first described PLRI as the result of LUCL insufficiency in 1991 [8], PLRI diagnosis has become more common [36] and various techniques for LCLC repair or reconstruction have been reported, as well as several modifications [2,17,36,37,41,43,44]. To the present day, there is no consensus on which treatment modality is more suitable for PLRI patients; nevertheless, some surgeons prefer arthroscopic techniques [3,17,41] and others open reconstruction [20,42].

For symptomatic patients with PLRI, surgical stabilization is recommended [20]. Regardless of the treatment method, the intention of re-stabilizing a joint is consistent; it aims to restore the form and functionality of the originally injured ligament. This study presents anatomical considerations for lateral-elbow-stabilizing structures, emphasizes the significance of the CEO in PLRI, and proposes a new treatment algorithm rooted in CEO integrity. The thought behind opting for arthroscopic LCL imbrication in patients with PLRI and either intact or moderately torn CEO is that open ligament reconstruction can be seen as an aggressive intervention, even for high-demand patients like professional athletes [29]. While open LUCL reconstructions provide impressive stability outcomes, the issues of extensive lateral soft tissue manipulations, scarring, and demanding postoperative rehabilitation protocols are noteworthy [3]. A well-known complication of LCL imbrication is subcutaneous irritation caused by suture knots [3], and suture sinking is recommended to decrease the irritation rate.

For patients suffering from partial CEO ruptures that are more extensive or complete ruptures without tendon retraction, isolated LCL imbrication may not prove sufficient.

Therefore, if the remaining soft tissue quality allows it, a more suitable option would be the plication reconstruction of LCLC [33]. The critical component is incorporating the CEO into the plicated soft tissue so it can be used to repair the ruptured extensors concurrently. In the augmentation process involving LCL imbrication, the anconeus is included in the construct, which enhances the tension of the lateral stabilizers [34]. The anconeus muscle mainly acts as an active posterolateral restraint rather than an active elbow extensor [28,30,45].

In cases involving PLRI and a fully ruptured and withdrawn CEO, the expected quality of the lateral structures' soft tissues is poor. This limits the possibilities for any soft tissue re-tensing procedures [10]. Furthermore, due to retraction, arthroscopic repair is not a viable option. Therefore, reconstructing the LUCL using an autograft seems to be a reliable alternative [2]. When it comes to graft fixation, careful consideration must be given to the isometric point on the humerus, the ulnar insertion point, and the appropriate graft tension to reduce the risk of failure [2,10]. The isometric point can be found using an anatomical and radiological method [2], and careful intraoperative testing of the expected graft tension is essential [10]. Importantly, the natural LUCL does not follow a straight line in three dimensions. Consequently, implanting a straight-lined graft may cause it to stretch and potentially jeopardize the reconstruction [39,40]. Furthermore, simultaneous osseous constraint lesions must also be properly addressed to reduce the risk of ligament reconstruction failure [10]. Although LUCL reconstruction with a tendon autograft restores the elbow's posterior lateral rotational stability, it does not always restore varus stability due to a potentially unchecked RCL dysfunction [39,40]. However, repairing the CEO after LUCL reconstruction may provide sufficient restoration of stability in varus [28].

The selection of the graft depends on the surgeon's preference. Autografts are superior to allografts, apart from donor-site morbidity [46]. Thus, it is essential that autograft harvesting is a feasible choice in the surgeon's armamentarium. Autograft options include the gracilis, the semitendinosus, the palmaris longus, the half-flexor carpi radialis, and the fascia lata, while all of them are strong enough to support the reconstruction [2,16,35,44]. It is the leading author's (C.K.) preference to harvest triceps tendon autografts. Postoperative stability rates are reported over 90% [39]. According to recently published data, recurrent instability ranges from 0 to 33% for LCL repair and reconstruction surgery [10]. Nevertheless, to our knowledge, there are no data regarding postoperative stability rates for LUCL reconstruction with triceps autografts in complete rupture with retraction of the CEO. Incorporating this algorithm into upcoming research protocols would have the potential to address this deficit in the existing literature.

The advancement in arthroscopic techniques in the upper limb offers substantial benefits to both the surgeon and the patient. Open procedures that address the lateral aspect of the elbow often fail to preserve the CEO, hindering shorter rehabilitation programs and delaying the return to work or sports [47]. By using arthroscopy, an all-round examination of the elbow joint can be performed before the main procedure. This method helps identify any concealed pathology [47]. While some researchers discourage arthroscopic treatment for elbow instability due to potential nerve damage (ulnar or radial) [47], a recent systematic review revealed that arthroscopic treatment yields equivalent outcomes to combined arthroscopy and open procedures, with fewer complications and minimal soft tissue injury [14]. This discovery is crucial, especially since a cadaveric study showed that the adverse effects of open techniques on the elbow, specifically regarding iatrogenic PLRI, are irreversible [38]. Therefore, managing PLRI through an open approach only seems beneficial when dealing with a CEO rupture with retraction.

Limitations of this study are present. Firstly, the accuracy of clinical tests to diagnose PLRI is patient- and examiner-dependent. This may lead to bias as minor instability might be underdiagnosed. However, in our proposed protocol, PLRI was confirmed by an arthroscope in all cases. There is no measurement of triceps brachii muscles preoperatively and before autografts are received, but the literature mentions no clinical reduction in muscle strength. Surgeons following this algorithm should be experienced arthroscopists. Another issue is the variability in the patient population and their demands. The postoperative protocol plays a significant role, and patient compliance can greatly affect the results. The primary limitation of this study is the lack of quantitative results. While our initial findings appear promising, the follow-up only extended to a maximum of 30 months. We would prefer to have a longer postoperative period for all participants before publishing the results. This would allow us to identify possible complications such as donor-site morbidity, the development of elbow arthritis, or a recurrence of instability. We advocate that arthroscopic surgeons use our treatment protocol on a larger scale as a tool for further research. It is not technically demanding for an experienced upper limb orthopedic surgeon and leverages existing knowledge. Multicenter studies could potentially uncover additional issues and suggest further improvements.

7. Conclusions

PLRI is a clinical entity that appears often in general practice, often masked under the veil of lateral epicondylitis. This treatment algorithm is intended for arthroscopic surgeons seeking to diagnose and treat an unstable elbow with as few complications as possible using minimally invasive techniques specific to each patient's condition. Based on the CEO's integrity, different techniques, or combinations thereof, may be applied, resorting to an open approach only in the most extreme cases where the CEO is completely torn and retracted (open LUCL reconstruction with graft). No or moderate lesions of the CEO could be treated with arthroscopic LCL imbrication, while extensive partial lesions or complete lesions without retraction of CEO are arthroscopically dealt with using plication and LCL imbrication. This proposed algorithm facilitates not only preoperative but also intraoperative planning with simultaneous avoidance of open surgery and possible complications. In every case, a preoperative MRI is mandatory to examine the CEO's integrity. Further research, including thorough follow-ups and optionally patient-reported outcome measure scores, is necessary.

Author Contributions: Conceptualization, C.K. and P.A.; methodology, C.K.; validation, K.B.; formal analysis, K.S.; investigation, A.T.; resources, M.K.; data curation, K.S.; writing—original draft preparation, M.K.; writing—review and editing, K.S.; supervision, F.M.; project administration, C.K. All authors have read and agreed to the published version of the manuscript.

Funding: This research received no external funding.

Institutional Review Board Statement: Not applicable.

Informed Consent Statement: Not applicable.

Data Availability Statement: No new data were created or analyzed in this study. Data sharing is not applicable to this article.

Conflicts of Interest: The authors declare no conflicts of interest.

References

1. Marinelli, A.; Graves, B.R.; Bain, G.I.; Pederzini, L. Treatment of elbow instability: State of the art. *J. ISAKOS* **2021**, *6*, 102–115. [CrossRef] [PubMed]
2. Carlier, Y.; Soubeyrand, M. Chronic elbow instability in adults: The why, when and how of ligament reconstruction. *Orthop. Traumatol. Surg. Res.* **2023**, *109*, 103449. [CrossRef] [PubMed]
3. Kohlprath, R.; Vuylsteke, K.; van Riet, R. Arthroscopic lateral collateral ligament imbrication of the elbow: Short-term clinical results. *J. Shoulder Elb. Surg.* **2022**, *31*, 2316–2321. [CrossRef] [PubMed]
4. Badhrinarayanan, S.; Desai, A.; Watson, J.J.; White, C.H.R.; Phadnis, J. Indications, Outcomes, and Complications of Lateral Ulnar Collateral Ligament Reconstruction of the Elbow for Chronic Posterolateral Rotatory Instability: A Systematic Review. *Am. J. Sports Med.* **2021**, *49*, 830–837. [CrossRef] [PubMed]
5. Amarasooriya, M.; Phadnis, J. Arthroscopic Diagnosis of Posterolateral Rotatory Instability of the Elbow. *Arthrosc. Tech.* **2020**, *9*, e1951–e1956. [CrossRef]
6. Noriego, D.; Carrera, A.; Tubbs, R.S.; Guibernau, J.; San Millán, M.; Iwanaga, J.; Cateura, A.; Sañudo, J.; Reina, F. The lateral ulnar collateral ligament: Anatomical and structural study for clinical application in the diagnosis and treatment of elbow lateral ligament injuries. *Clin. Anat.* **2023**, *36*, 866–874. [CrossRef] [PubMed]

7. O'Driscoll, S.W.; Morrey, B.F.; Korinek, S.; An, K.N. Elbow subluxation and dislocation. A spectrum of instability. *Clin. OrthopRelat Res.* **1992**, *280*, 186–197. [PubMed]
8. O'Driscoll, S.W.; Bell, D.F.; Morrey, B.F. Posterolateral rotatory instability of the elbow. *J. Bone Jt. Surg. Am.* **1991**, *73*, 440–446. [CrossRef] [PubMed]
9. Arrigoni, P.; Cucchi, D.; D'Ambrosi, R.; Butt, U.; Safran, M.R.; Denard, P.; Randelli, P. Intra-articular findings in symptomatic minor instability of the lateral elbow (SMILE). *Knee Surg. Sports Traumatol. Arthrosc.* **2017**, *25*, 2255–2263. [CrossRef] [PubMed]
10. O'Driscoll, S.W.; Chaney, G.K. Preoperative and operative risk factors for failed lateral collateral ligament reconstruction. *JSES Int.* **2023**, *7*, 2578–2586. [CrossRef]
11. Dunning, C.E.; Zarzour, Z.D.; Patterson, S.D.; Johnson, J.A.; King, G.J. Ligamentous stabilizers against posterolateral rotatory instability of the elbow. *J. Bone Jt. Surg. Am.* **2001**, *83*, 1823–1828. [CrossRef] [PubMed]
12. Imatani, J.; Ogura, T.; Morito, Y.; Hashizume, H.; Inoue, H. Anatomic and histologic studies of lateral collateral ligament complex of the elbow joint. *J. Shoulder Elb. Surg.* **1999**, *8*, 625–627. [CrossRef] [PubMed]
13. Anakwenze, O.A.; Kwon, D.; O'Donnell, E.; Levine, W.N.; Ahmad, C.S. Surgical treatment of posterolateral rotatory instability of the elbow. *Arthrosc. J. Arthrosc. Relat. Surg.* **2014**, *30*, 866–871. [CrossRef] [PubMed]
14. Goodwin, D.; Dynin, M.; MacDonnell, J.R.; Kessler, M.W. The role of arthroscopy in chronic elbow instability. *Arthrosc. J. Arthrosc. Relat. Surg.* **2013**, *29*, 2029–2036. [CrossRef] [PubMed]
15. Scheiderer, B.; Imhoff, F.B.; Kia, C.; Aglio, J.; Morikawa, D.; Obopilwe, E.; Cote, M.P.; Lacheta, L.; Imhoff, A.B.; Mazzocca, A.D.; et al. LUCL internal bracing restores posterolateral rotatory stability of the elbow. *Knee Surg. Sports Traumatol. Arthrosc.* **2020**, *28*, 1195–1201. [CrossRef] [PubMed]
16. Conti Mica, M.; Caekebeke, P.; van Riet, R. Lateral collateral ligament injuries of the elbow—*Chronic* posterolateral rotatory instability (PLRI). *EFORT Open Rev.* **2017**, *1*, 461–468. [CrossRef] [PubMed]
17. Sachinis, N.P.; Yiannakopoulos, C.K.; Beitzel, K.; Koukos, C. Arthroscopic Modified Elbow Lateral Collateral Ligament Imbrication: An Operative Technique. *Arthrosc. Tech.* **2023**, *12*, e709–e714. [CrossRef] [PubMed]
18. Baron, J.E.; Shamrock, A.G.; Wolf, B.R. Posterolateral Rotary Instability of the Elbow in Adolescents: A Report of 2 Cases and Review of the Literature. *JBJS Case Connect.* **2019**, *9*, e0504. [CrossRef] [PubMed]
19. Kholinne, E.; Liu, H.; Kim, H.; Kwak, J.M.; Koh, K.H.; Jeon, I.H. Systematic Review of Elbow Instability in Association With Refractory Lateral Epicondylitis: Myth or Fact? *Am. J. Sports Med.* **2021**, *49*, 2542–2550. [CrossRef] [PubMed]
20. Schneider, M.M.; Müller, K.; Hollinger, B.; Nietschke, R.; Zimmerer, A.; Ries, C.; Burkhart, K.J. Lateral Ulnar Collateral Ligament Reconstruction for Posterolateral Rotatory Instability after Failed Common Extensor Origin Release: Outcomes at Minimum 2-Year Follow-up. *Orthop. J. Sports Med.* **2022**, *10*, 23259671211069340. [CrossRef]
21. Schnetzke, M.; Ellwein, A.; Maier, D.; Wagner, F.C.; Grützner, P.A.; Guehring, T. Injury patterns following simple elbow dislocation: Radiological analysis implies existence of a pure valgus dislocation mechanism. *Arch. Orthop. Trauma Surg.* **2021**, *141*, 1649–1657. [CrossRef] [PubMed]
22. Kim, Y.S.; Kim, S.T.; Lee, K.H.; Ahn, J.M.; Gong, H.S. Radiocapitellar incongruity of the radial head in magnetic resonance imaging correlates with pathologic changes of the lateral elbow stabilizers in lateral epicondylitis. *PLoS ONE* **2021**, *16*, e0254037. [CrossRef] [PubMed]
23. Jeon, J.Y.; Lee, M.H.; Jeon, I.H.; Chung, H.W.; Lee, S.H.; Shin, M.J. Lateral epicondylitis: Associations of MR imaging and clinical assessments with treatment options in patients receiving conservative and arthroscopic managements. *Eur. Radiol.* **2018**, *28*, 972–981. [CrossRef] [PubMed]
24. Fedorka, C.J.; Oh, L.S. Posterolateral rotatory instability of the elbow. *Curr. Rev. Musculoskelet. Med.* **2016**, *9*, 240–246. [CrossRef] [PubMed]
25. Seki, A.; Olsen, B.S.; Jensen, S.L.; Eygendaal, D.; Søjbjerg, J.O. Functional anatomy of the lateral collateral ligament complex of the elbow: Configuration of Y and its role. *J. Shoulder Elb. Surg.* **2002**, *11*, 53–59. [CrossRef] [PubMed]
26. Mehta, J.A.; Bain, G.I. Posterolateral rotatory instability of the elbow. *J. Am. Acad. Orthop. Surg.* **2004**, *12*, 405–415. [CrossRef] [PubMed]
27. Regan, W.; Lapner, P.C. Prospective evaluation of two diagnostic apprehension signs for posterolateral instability of the elbow. *J. Shoulder Elb. Surg.* **2006**, *15*, 344–346. [CrossRef] [PubMed]
28. Hackl, M.; Wegmann, K.; Ries, C.; Leschinger, T.; Burkhart, K.J.; Müller, L.P. Reliability of Magnetic Resonance Imaging Signs of Posterolateral Rotatory Instability of the Elbow. *J. Hand Surg. Am.* **2015**, *40*, 1428–1433. [CrossRef] [PubMed]
29. Pierreux, P.; Caekebeke, P.; van Riet, R. The role of arthroscopy in instability of the elbow. *JSES Int.* **2022**, *7*, 2594–2599. [CrossRef]
30. Mahasupachai, N.; Samathi, N.; Premsiri, A.; Chanlalit, C. The sonographic posterolateral rotatory stress test: Normal ulnohumeral gap difference in healthy volunteers. *J. Orthop. Surg.* **2022**, *30*, 1–7. [CrossRef]
31. Walz, D.M.; Newman, J.S.; Konin, G.P.; Ross, G. Epicondylitis: Pathogenesis, imaging, and treatment. *Radiographics* **2010**, *30*, 167–184. [CrossRef] [PubMed]
32. Bredella, M.A.; Tirman, P.F.; Fritz, R.C.; Feller, J.F.; Wischer, T.K.; Genant, H.K. MR imaging findings of lateral ulnar collateral ligament abnormalities in patients with lateral epicondylitis. *AJR Am. J. Roentgenol.* **1999**, *173*, 1379–1382. [CrossRef] [PubMed]
33. Savoie, F.H., 3rd; Field, L.D.; Gurley, D.J. Arthroscopic and open radial ulnohumeral ligament reconstruction for posterolateral rotatory instability of the elbow. *Hand Clin.* **2009**, *25*, 323–329. [CrossRef] [PubMed]

34. Badre, A.; Axford, D.T.; Banayan, S.; Johnson, J.A.; King, G.J.W. Role of the anconeus in the stability of a lateral ligament and common extensor origin-deficient elbow: An in vitro biomechanical study. *J. Shoulder Elb. Surg.* **2019**, *28*, 974–981. [CrossRef] [PubMed]
35. Baker, C.L., Jr.; Murphy, K.P.; Gottlob, C.A.; Curd, D.T. Arthroscopic classification and treatment of lateral epicondylitis: Two-year clinical results. *J. Shoulder Elb. Surg.* **2000**, *9*, 475–482. [CrossRef] [PubMed]
36. Savoie, F.H., 3rd; O'Brien, M.J.; Field, L.D.; Gurley, D.J. Arthroscopic and open radial ulnohumeral ligament reconstruction for posterolateral rotatory instability of the elbow. *Clin. Sports Med.* **2010**, *29*, 611–618. [CrossRef] [PubMed]
37. Caekebeke, P.; Mica, M.A.C.; van Riet, R. Evaluation and Management of Posterolateral Rotatory Instability (PLRI). In *The Unstable Elbow*; Tashjian, R., Ed.; Springer: Cham, Switzerland, 2017. [CrossRef]
38. Daniels, S.D.; France, T.J.; Peek, K.J.; Tucker, N.J.; Baldini, T.; Catalano, L.W.; Lauder, A. Posterolateral Rotatory Instability Develops Following the Modified Kocher Approach and Does Not Resolve Following Interval Repair. *J. Bone Jt. Surg. Am.* **2023**, *105*, 1601–1610. [CrossRef] [PubMed]
39. Schoch, C.; Dittrich, M.; Seilern Und Aspang, J.; Geyer, M.; Geyer, S. Autologous triceps tendon graft for LUCL reconstruction of the elbow: Clinical outcome after 7.5 years. *Eur. J. Orthop. Surg. Traumatol.* **2022**, *32*, 1111–1118. [CrossRef] [PubMed]
40. Dehlinger, F.; Ries, C.; Hollinger, B. LUCL-Bandplastik mit Trizepssehnentransplantat zur Therapie der posterolateralen Rotationsinstabilität am Ellenbogen. *Oper. Orthop. Traumatol.* **2014**, *26*, 414–429. [CrossRef] [PubMed]
41. Chanlalit, C.; Mahasupachai, N.; Sakdapanichkul, C. Arthroscopic lateral collateral ligament imbrication for treatment of atraumatic posterolateral rotatory instability. *J. Orthop. Surg.* **2022**, *30*, 1–7. [CrossRef]
42. Lannes, X.; Traverso, A.; Wehrli, L.; Goetti, P. Douleurs latérales du coude chez l'adulte: Algorithme de prise en charge [Support algorithm for lateral elbow pain syndrome in adults]. *Rev. Med. Suisse* **2023**, *19*, 2336–2343. (In French) [CrossRef] [PubMed]
43. Eigenschink, M.; Pauzenberger, L.; Laky, B.; Ostermann, R.C.; Anderl, W.; Heuberer, P.R. Lateral ulnar collateral ligament reconstruction using an autologous triceps tendon graft for subclinical posterolateral rotatory instability in recalcitrant lateral epicondylitis. *J. Shoulder Elb. Surg.* **2023**, *32*, 1262–1270. [CrossRef] [PubMed]
44. Tranier, M.; Bacle, G.; Marteau, E.; Sos, C.; Laulan, J.; Roulet, S. Lateral elbow ligament reconstruction for posterolateral rotatory instability: 10 years follow-up in 32 patients. *JSES Int.* **2022**, *7*, 357–363. [CrossRef] [PubMed]
45. Pereira, B.P. Revisiting the anatomy and biomechanics of the anconeus muscle and its role in elbow stability. *Ann. Anat.* **2013**, *195*, 365–370. [CrossRef] [PubMed]
46. Delgove, A.; Weigert, R.; Casoli, V. Evaluation of donor site morbidity after medial triceps brachii free flap for lower limb reconstruction. *Arch. Orthop. Trauma Surg.* **2017**, *137*, 1659–1666. [CrossRef] [PubMed]
47. Chow, H.Y.; Eygendaal, D.; The, B. Elbow arthroscopy—Indications and technique. *J. Clin. Orthop. Trauma* **2021**, *19*, 147–153. [CrossRef] [PubMed]

Journal of
Clinical Medicine

MDPI

Brief Report

Case Studies of a Simulation Workflow to Improve Bone Healing Assessment in Impending Non-Unions

Tanja C. Maisenbacher [1], Saskia Libicher [1], Felix Erne [1], Maximilian M. Menger [1], Marie K. Reumann [1], Yannick Schindler [2], Frank Niemeyer [2], Lucas Engelhardt [2], Tina Histing [1] and Benedikt J. Braun [1,*]

1 Department of Trauma and Reconstructive Surgery, Eberhard Karls University Tuebingen, BG Klinik Tuebingen, 72076 Tuebingen, Germany; tmaisenbacher@bgu-tuebingen.de (T.C.M.); slibicher@bgu-tuebingen.de (S.L.); ferne@bgu-tuebingen.de (F.E.); mmenger@bgu-tuebingen.de (M.M.M.); mreumann@bgu-tuebingen.de (M.K.R.); thisting@bgu-tuebingen.de (T.H.)

2 Project Team OSORA—Medical Fracture Analytics, Ulm University, Helmholtzstr. 20, 89081 Ulm, Germany; yannick.schindler@osora.de (Y.S.); frank.niemeyer@osora.de (F.N.); publication@lucasengelhardt.de (L.E.)

* Correspondence: bbraun@bgu-tuebingen.de; Tel.: +49-7071-606-1164

Abstract: Background: The healing potential of a fracture is determined by mechanical and biological factors. Simulation-based workflows can help assess these factors to assist in predicting non-unions. The aim of this study was the introduction of two use cases for a novel patient-specific simulation workflow based on clinically available information. **Methods:** The used software is an extension of the "Ulm Bone Healing model" and was applied in two cases with non-union development after fracture fixation to show its principal feasibility. The clinical and radiographic information, starting from initial treatment, were used to feed the simulation process. **Results:** The simulation predicted non-union development and axial deviation in a mechanically driven non-union. In the case of a biological non-union, a slow, incomplete healing course was correctly identified. However, the time offset in callus bridging was discordant between the simulation and the distinctly slower healing response in the clinical case. **Conclusions**: The simulation workflow presented in the two clinical use cases allowed for the identification of fractures at risk for impending non-union immediately after the initial fixation based on available clinical and radiographic information. Further validation in a large non-union cohort is needed to increase the model's precision, especially in biologically challenging cases, and show its validity as a screening instrument.

Keywords: fracture healing; non-union; mal-union; individualized; simulation; vascularization; biomechanics

1. Introduction

Despite substantial research and progress concerning fracture treatment and healing, non-union still occurs in about 5–10% of all fracture cases [1]. Depending on the fracture location and surrounding conditions, the rates can increase to up to 20% [2]. Major risk factors include open fractures and high degrees of soft tissue injury in terms of biological factors, and stability as well as the osteosynthetic construct setup, in terms of mechanical factors [3–6]. Due to long healing periods, non-union treatment not only poses a substantial socioeconomic impact on healthcare systems but also has a significant effect on health-related quality of life concerning both physical and mental health [7,8]. The diagnosis of fracture non-union is commonly a multistage process: Pain and loss of function are the first clinical symptoms driving further analysis. Radiological diagnostics by X-ray and computed tomography (CT) confirm failure or delay of fracture healing. Deciding on when a non-union is established and needs further revision requires a high degree of expertise and is subject to the timing associated with diagnostics [9]. There is still no score or gold standard guidelines universally agreed upon concerning the diagnosis of a non-union, further complicating its treatment and timing in clinical practice [10–14]. In particular, in the early phases of healing, adequate fracture healing monitoring is challenging [15]. Thus, identifying a non-union adequately often takes up to 6–9 months, potentially delaying the initiation of revision therapy [2].

Fracture healing after fixation is driven by both mechanical and vascularity-associated factors. Mechanical conditions in the fracture gap depend on the type of osteosynthesis, the fracture morphology, and patient loading [16]. Claes et al. defined experimental healing boundary conditions and hypothesized two major mechanical influences: relative strain and hydrostatic pressure [17]. Both underly and influence the dynamics of the bone healing process. Secondary bone healing is characterized by different stages [18]. The inflammation stage is characterized by hematoma and the infiltration of different cell types and growth factors like bone morphogenetic proteins. The formation of a soft callus by endochondral ossification and replacement by a hard callus afterward is followed by the final stage of bone healing and bone remodeling, leading to the recovery of the lamellar bone to the state before the fracture. Stiffness and loading define interfragmentary strain and thus cell differentiation. Additionally, adequate vascularization is essential to supply the fracture site with sufficient oxygenation and growth factors [19]. Insufficient blood supply can be related to patient risk factors such as diabetes and nicotine abuse, as well as injury- and surgery-related factors, such as open fractures or the surgical approach [2].

In principle, numerical simulations can predict and visualize the fracture healing process, and these techniques have already been applied to limited case series in clinical settings. Their main limitation is the degree of precision given in their healing assessment, largely influenced by the number of input parameters used for the simulation [20]. Combining motion-capturing data to define individual loading and radiological data, it was possible to simulate the mechanical fracture environment in patients with tibial non-union [21]. By mapping interfragmentary strain and the von Mises stress distribution within different points of the fracture gap, the healing potential of a lower leg fracture situation can be predicted based on individual loading characteristics, gait speeds, and fracture geometry [21,22]. The principal feasibility of this technique has since been shown in other fracture and non-union situations both in the upper and lower extremity [2]. Many of these models are driven by motion capturing and are aimed at either mechanics or biology. Based on the Ulm Bone Healing model, software was developed that allowed for the simulation of the healing process of different fracture situations using both mechanical and clinical input, taken only from clinical imaging and history [23,24]. Thus far, this model has been used to simulate the healing process in various experimental scenarios in sheep, as well as in the human tibia and the distal radius. Recently, the algorithm was applied to human femoral shaft fractures, where it was able to accurately predict the healing potential and clinical course [25]. While the principal detection capability of the simulation workflow in femoral fractures, including non-union cases, was shown, a further more detailed analysis of the concept's feasibility in dedicated, challenging healing situations is needed [25].

The aim of the present study was to introduce two use cases of an adapted simulation workflow based on the Ulm Bone Healing model in impending non-unions of the lower extremity and highlight its strengths and weaknesses to detect healing disturbance both in mechanically and biologically challenging cases.

2. Materials and Methods

Principal ethical approval was obtained from the ethical committee of Tuebingen University (application number 318/2022BO2, 840/2019B02, 13 July 2022). Informed consent including the use of patient data for analysis and publication, anonymization and secure data storage, the potential data safety risks, and patients' right to withdraw consent was given by both patients to participate in the collection of movement data and the fracture and non-union simulation based on their clinical and imaging data. As a feasibility study, we aimed to highlight the workflow's general applicability in two challenging cases, one mechanically and one biologically driven, to provide a foundation for emerging systematic research. Both patients were consecutively enrolled after the availability of the simulation workflow at our center. Additional consent was given to share the data with the simulation provider in a pseudonymized fashion over a DSGVO conform server. We followed the Danish Orthopaedic Trauma Society's definition of a non-union for this article, where a fracture that will not heal without further intervention is considered a non-union [11]. A fracture that is delayed beyond the expected healing course is considered a delayed union.

2.1. Case Data

The first case is a 54-year-old healthy patient suffering from a closed tibial shaft fracture (AO/OTA 42B3c) and a distal fibular fracture (Figure 1) after being hit by a tree. The closed lower leg fracture was immediately addressed by internal nail fixation of the tibia and an open reduction procedure of the distal fibula with plate osteosynthesis at an external institution. Two months later, the patient was admitted to our clinic due to ongoing pain and increasing axial deviation. The CT scan showed an axial deviation of the tibia and fibula. A two-staged revision was performed due to the slow healing of the fibular-sided incision. The wound was excised, and the plate was removed during the first step. No bacterial contamination was detected. One week later, exchange nailing with reaming was performed. The patient was changed from a 9 mm to a 10 mm diameter nail. Axis deviation was corrected with percutaneously placed blocking screws distally both in ap and mediolateral directions. Postoperatively, the patient was immediately prescribed full weight-bearing. Seven months later, complete fracture healing was documented (Figure 1).

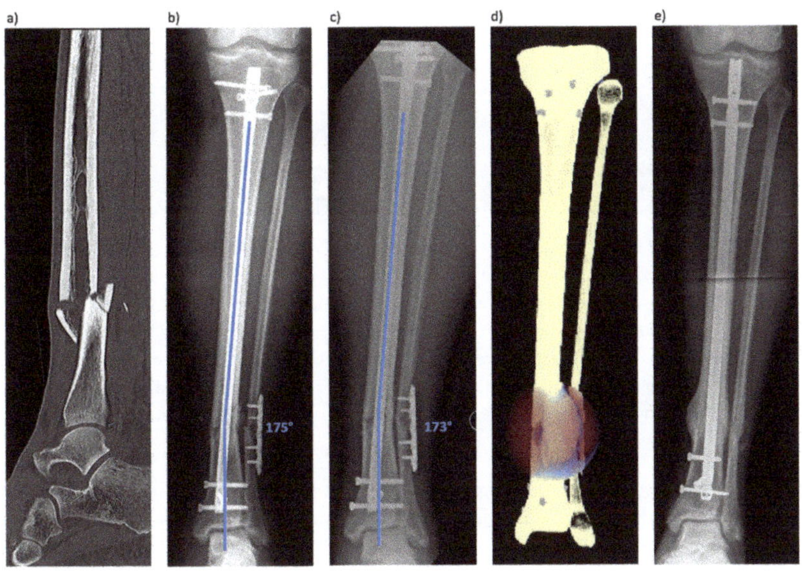

Figure 1. (**a**) Lateral CT image of the lower leg fracture (AO/OTA 42B3c). (**b**) Ap (anteroposterior) radiograph taken one day after initial surgery. The tibial fracture was addressed by nailing and the fibula fracture by plate osteosynthesis. (**c**) Ap radiograph taken 3 weeks after the initial surgery showed progressive loss of reduction and no signs of healing. (**d**) The simulation results at the final timepoint with secondary dislocation in accordance with the clinical result and tissue differentiation is shown for the 100% body weight weight-bearing scenario (brown-red = connective tissue, blue = cartilage, light orange = woven bone, light yellow = lamellar bone). (**e**) Ap radiograph taken about 6 months post-revision surgery showing timely consolidation and correction of leg axis.

The second case is a 55-year-old patient with a closed femoral shaft fracture (AO/OTA 32B2b) (Figure 2). The patient suffered from cardiovascular disease with previous stent implantation, high blood pressure, and gastroesophageal reflux disease. His regularly taken medication was aspirin, bisoprolol, and rosuvastatin. He was treated at an external institution with antegrade femoral nailing. An additional lateral incision was performed to openly reduce an interposed fracture fragment, and the fracture hematoma was rinsed out as per the surgical report. Five months after the initial treatment, the patient came to our clinic due to ongoing pain at the former fracture site and persisting inability to bear weight on the extremity. The CT scan showed delayed fracture healing with no callus formation and visible fracture gaps. Based on the history and clinical imaging, the non-union was deemed to be primarily of biological cause, so 3 weeks later, the patient underwent revision surgery with reamed exchange nailing. The patient was changed from a 9 mm to a 12 mm diameter nail. Immediate full weight-bearing was prescribed postoperatively. Seven months later, the patient declared to have no more pain, and the conventional radiograph, as well as the CT scan, showed sufficient callus formation and fracture healing (Figure 2).

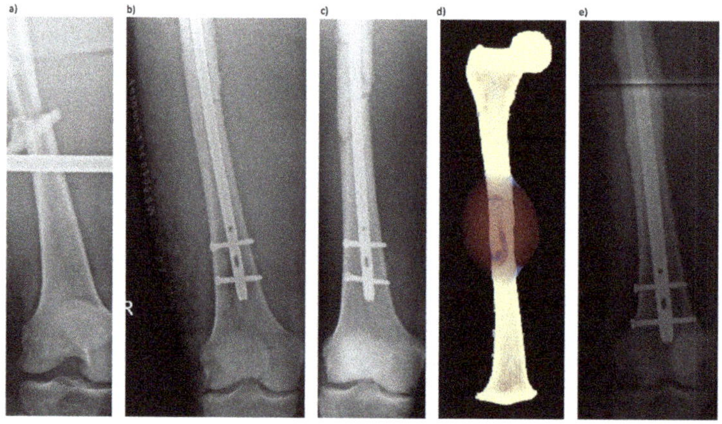

Figure 2. (**a**) Ap radiograph of the dislocated femur fracture (AO/OTA 32B2b). (**b**) Ap radiograph showing the initial nail osteosynthesis one day after surgery with the large lateral-based incision used for the open reduction procedure of the intercalary fragment. (**c**) Four months after trauma, no consolidation or callus formation was observed in the radiograph. (**d**) The simulation results at the final timepoint with tissue differentiation are shown for the 5% body weight weight-bearing scenario (brown-red = connective tissue, blue = cartilage, light orange = woven bone, light yellow = lamellar bone). (**e**) Ap radiograph taken about 5 months post-revision surgery showing timely consolidation.

2.2. *Digital Twin of the Fracture Situation*

The Ulm tissue-level bone healing model predicts the evolution of different tissues, woven and lamellar bone, fibrocartilage, and fibrous connective tissue, throughout fracture healing [23,24,26]. Both mechanical and biological stimuli are taken into consideration. The simulation is based on established biomechanical observations and the mechano-regulating hypothesis by Claes and Heigele [27,28]. Distortional and dilatational strains have been identified to be determining mechanical factors for tissue differentiation and remodeling [26]. In addition, biological parameters like the physiological condition of the tissue surrounding the fracture and vascularization were considered in the simulation by using fuzzy logic rules. The current strain at every point of the healing process was analyzed by the finite element method (Ansys® Mechanical APDL, Version 2020 R2; Ansys, Inc., Canonsburg, PA, USA). The presented model was therefore able to predict the development of the different tissue types over time and the time till fracture consolidation. The simulation of bone healing was applied for 240 days, and the simulated healing process was then compared to the original outcome. The time of consolidation was derived automatically from the primary simulation results using a path-search algorithm to detect connections of lamellar bone in all four quadrants of the bone. If the simulation predicted bony bridging in at least three quadrants within the simulated days, the case was classified as "union"; otherwise, the case was classified as a "non-union". A detailed description of the general simulation workflow can be found in recent publications [23,24], and it was clinically applied to femoral fractures in the study by Degenhart et al. [25].

2.3. Application to the Clinical Cases

To simulate the healing process, the first step was to create a finite element model of the individual bone anatomy, fracture, and osteosynthesis of the patient based on the provided CT scans in order to reconstruct the postoperative situation. For each of the cases, 3D Slicer [29] was used to segment the tibia/fibula or the femur, respectively, as well as the implant from the CT image data. This step enabled the generation of an accurate three-dimensional (3D) geometric representation of the fractured bone. Since the CT scans were not taken immediately after the surgery but at a later time, we manually realigned the fragments based on the postoperative X-ray scans.

The fracture area was augmented with a so-called "healing domain" that encompassed the entire fractured area, representing the area in the immediate vicinity of the fracture where we expected tissue formation/differentiation due to mechanical and biological stimuli to take place, according to our tissue differentiation algorithm. The geometries were discretized into finite elements using appropriate meshing techniques (Ansys® Mechanical APDL, Version 2020 R2; Ansys, Inc., Canonsburg, PA, USA). For the initial tissue composition, we assumed that the cortical and cancellous bone consisted of 100% lamellar fully vascularized bone, while the remaining tissue (in between and proximally to the fracture) was assumed to consist of initially avascular soft tissue.

To determine the loading conditions, the relevant literature on physiological loading scenarios for femoral and tibia fractures was consulted. These loading conditions were then applied to the FE model to simulate the mechanical response of the fractured bone. In both cases, the patients were assumed to bear full weight after surgery. According to our recent study with femur fractures [25], the maximum load occurring during the normal gait cycle was assumed. Therefore, the muscle and joint loading conditions, as stated by Heller et al. (2005) [30], were used, which allowed us to express loading in terms of the percentage of patients' body weight. The tibia case was loaded as described by Zhao et al. by applying a 55/45% split of the peak load during the gait cycle (2.2 times the body weight) on the medial and lateral compartments of the tibial plateau [31].

Using the reconstructed geometry and the patient's weight, the simulations were able to be performed within 24 h of simulation time on a high-performance workstation (AMD Ryzen 5900X, 128 GB RAM, AMD, Santa Clara, CA, USA). See Supplementary Materials for more details.

3. Results

3.1. Patient 1 (Tibial Fracture)

The fracture healing simulation for this patient revealed that this fracture was not going to unite. During the 240 simulation days, cortical bridging was never seen for more than two cortices (Figure 3). Additionally, the simulation showed a deviation of the fibular axis throughout the healing process, in line with the clinical presentation of an increasing leg axis deviation before revision.

3.2. Patient 2 (Femoral Fracture)

Assuming an immediate full weight-bearing state, the fracture healing simulation for this patient concluded that this fracture was going to unite. During the 240 simulation days, cortical bridging was seen in this patient for three out of the four cortices after 184 days. The anterior cortex did not show bone healing within this period (Figure 4). Calculations with lower levels of weight-bearing in the region of 5–10% of the patient's body weight, in line with the clinical situation, resulted in the correct prediction of non-union development with the progressive dissipation of the interposed fragment (Figure 4).

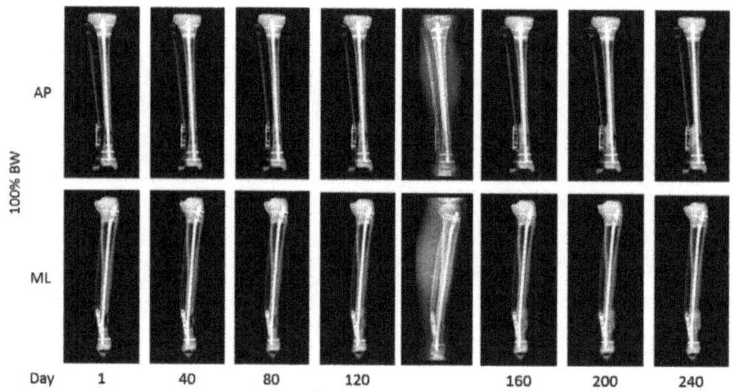

Figure 3. Fracture healing simulation assuming the full weight-bearing of the patient. The simulation shows the failure of the union of the fracture with progressive axial deviation. Simulated radiographs are shown for selected days after the initial surgery (1, 40, 80, 120, 160, 200, and 240 days after surgery) in an ap (**top row**) and lateral projection (ML, mediolateral) (**bottom row**). After day 120, a clinically matched actual lower leg radiograph before the revision is shown.

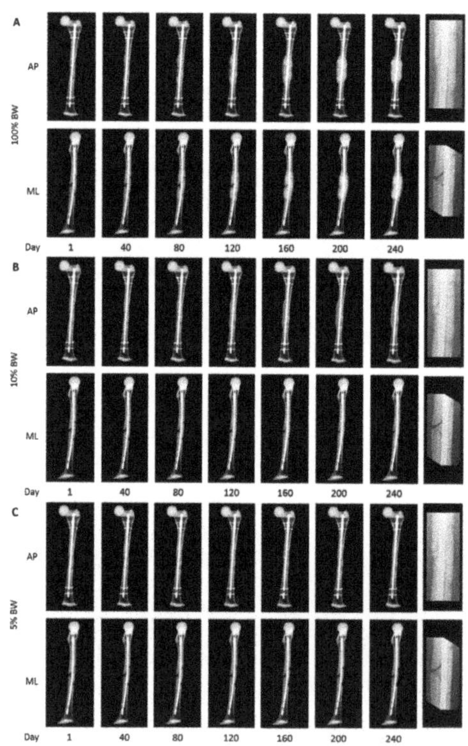

Figure 4. (**A**) Simulation of fracture healing according to full weight-bearing during 240 days. This simulation shows a slow fracture healing with cortical bridging of 3 out of 4 cortices after 184 days. (**B**) This simulation shows the fracture healing assuming a weight-bearing state of 10% of body weight. Here, no consolidation could be observed, and less callus formation occurred. (**C**) Simulation of fracture healing assuming a weight-bearing state of 5% of body weight. Again, no fracture healing is shown with a continuously atrophic intercalary fracture fragment. After day 240, for each series, a clinically matched actual radiograph focused on the callus situation before the revision is shown.

4. Discussion

The present study shows two use cases of a simulation workflow based on the Ulm Bone Healing Model to analyze the healing course of challenging fractures progressing to non-unions. The model was able to determine the impending non-union in a mechanically challenging fracture case and also the increasing axial deviation that occurred during the initial treatment aftercare. Furthermore, the simulation of a mainly biologically driven non-union identified its slow healing course while also highlighting the system's limitations pertaining to individual patient weight-bearing. The current work shows the opportunities as well as pitfalls associated with this technique.

Determining the healing potential of fractures, especially during the early treatment course, remains challenging under clinical conditions, thus often leading to a significant delay in the diagnosis of a fracture non-union [2]. In particular, the biological viability of the patient and fracture situation is difficult to assess in all detail, as well as the interaction of mechanics, biology, and the individual situation of each patient according to, e.g., surgical treatment, and compliance. Several clinical scores have aimed at determining the risk for non-union early during the treatment of a lower extremity fracture, most prominently the Non-Union Risk Development Score [32]. While this score gives an estimation of the risk of healing delay, it only incorporates simple clinical information, without fracture mechanics or osteosynthetic construct, thus leaving a degree of imprecision, which makes it more of a general risk assessment tool to identify patients at higher risk for non-union. Chloros and colleagues have recently looked at the four most common clinical scoring systems, namely the Leeds–Genoa Non-Union Index (LEG-NUI), the NURD, the FRACTING score, and the Tibial Fracture Healing Score (TFHS) [33]. They have shown high positive and negative predictive values, especially for the LEG-NUI score, in a retrospective application to tibial non-union cases. An advantage of these scoring systems is that they can be applied during the first 6–12 weeks of clinical treatment and are based on clinical information. As part of their conclusion, the authors advise that further prospective studies are needed to provide more evidence regarding the scores' useability and predictability. Another clinically applicable prediction method to determine the fracture healing potential is radiographically [34]. Different scores have been described for both the upper and lower extremity most prominently for tibial (Radiographic Union Score Tibia (RUST) and modified RUST (mRUST)), femoral (Radiographic Union Score Hip (RUSH)) and humerus (Radiographic Union Score Humerus (RUSHU)). While these scores greatly improve interrater reliability, only limited evidence exists regarding cut-off values and their prospective use.

In an attempt to increase the level of detail in assessing the healing potential of a fracture situation, different simulation models have been established and used in clinical settings. Dailey and colleagues have described a simulation approach based on low-dose CT imaging data that were used for virtual mechanical testing and provided a structural callus assessment to predict time to union and enable the early diagnosis of compromised healing, as early as 12 weeks after a fracture [35]. Other research groups have described further healing simulations based on motion capturing and ground reaction data in conjunction with patient imaging to determine the interfragmentary strain of fractures and non-unions [22]. They were able to determine the influence of different mechanical parameters, such as weight-bearing, gait speed, and the overall setup of the osteosynthetic construct, on the healing chances of a fracture. However, these simulations are based on additional information that goes beyond routinely available clinical data and primarily focus on fracture mechanics. Few simulations in a clinical situation have already employed a combined biological and mechanical simulation approach [23–25].

The results of the simulation of patient 1 highlight the system's principal capability to assess the mechanical situation based solely on available clinical information. It was able to determine that this fracture would not heal and that the leg axis deviation, which was also encountered during the clinical course, would increase. The precision and capability of a mechanical-based fracture simulation in non-union cases to determine the risk of implant failure and healing delay have already been reported by other groups [22]. However, many of these systems are based on additional information and sensors, such as inertial measurement units or the ground reaction force, limiting their general clinical applicability. The workflow presented here is based only on clinical and imaging information obtained during standard-of-care treatment without additional measures.

The results of the second patient highlight both the opportunities and shortcomings of the presented workflow in a challenging biological situation. The mechanical setup of the initial treatment was sound with good reduction and intramedullary nail osteosynthesis with good sufficient nail fit, well within accepted ranges [36]. Accordingly, the mechanics during the simulation were seen as adequate. Moreover, assuming immediate full weight-bearing, in this case, would have led to the algorithm assuming a slow but complete fracture healing, with cortical bridging on three sides after a little over 180 days. This did completely change in weight-bearing simulation scenarios equivalent to 5–10% body weight. Here, no healing within the simulation timeframe of 240 days was seen in accordance with the clinical course. The patient's fracture did not exhibit adequate healing response at 5 months with severely limited function and mobility due to continuing pain at the non-union site. At the request of the patient, the decision was made to revise the non-union with an exchange nailing procedure, and subsequent fracture healing was observed. So, despite the very slow healing course predicted in a full weight-bearing scenario, a different healing outcome was obtained clinically. Only significantly adapting the weight-bearing condition led to the correct prediction. This outlines the need for adequate monitoring of the patient and adapting the simulation to the patient's individual capability of weight-bearing and again shows the system's capability for the correct prediction of the mechanical situation without the need for additional data apart from routine control imaging. If full weight-bearing is not possible, a different mechanical impact on the fracture site has to be assumed. Understandably, the simulation can only assess the biological parameters included in the available clinical input data. Without knowing the surgical report of the initial treatment performed at an outside institution, the real extent of surgical tissue damage cannot be identified by clinical and imaging data alone. During the treatment, the large intercalary fragment was completely removed, reinserted, and openly reduced during nail passage, potentially devascularizing large portions of the fracture situation. The system only considers clinical information and imaging, not taking into account the patient's decreased biological state due to the additional surgical trauma. Future versions of the simulation can certainly be adapted to incorporate these biological healing challenges in more detail.

As opposed to other simulation techniques, in fracture non-union, mainly focusing on individual fracture mechanics, the current approach also incorporates biological aspects through routinely available data. This underlines the system's potentially broad applicability in all clinical settings and beyond specialized study centers and lab situations. The information for the clinical course and the risk for delayed healing can be assessed immediately after the initial fracture treatment, allowing for the identification of patients at risk for delayed healing who require a closer observation early on. The time taken for the simulation algorithm is clinically feasible and took about 48 h per case for the current analysis. As the simulation is based on readily available clinical information, the main cost driver is the cost of personnel to set up and run the simulation. This is certainly a limitation compared to clinical scoring systems with comparable early applicability and without the associated cost. Future hardware and software developments will likely increase the speed and precision of the simulation workflow significantly, further increasing its clinical usefulness. Integration into the clinical information system could help provide a simulation with minimal a number of physician and patient input. Certainly, further studies are needed to refine the workflow's detection capability and predictive precision.

Provided further validation of the workflow shows its continued precision along the lines of the results presented here, the earlier detection of fractures at risk for a healing delay has several potential benefits addressing both the patient's individual, as well as socioeconomic burden of disease [28]. On the patient side, early interventions ranging from adaptation of the aftercare regime to surgical treatment are possible. As intramedullary nailing usually entails full weight-bearing, potential adaptations can be to reduce weight-bearing in situations with increased interfragmentary motion, while the frequency and intensity of a full weight-bearing state can be addressed in understimulated situations (e.g., climbing stairs or rising from the chair leads to a reaction force much higher than walking in a straight line) [14,15,21]. If the simulation determines that healing cannot be achieved by modulation of the weight-bearing input, the stiffness of the osteosynthesis construct can be adjusted: Dynamization, reverse dynamization, and augmentative plating, as well as exchange nailing, to optimize nail fit are all potential options that could be simulated before surgery and scaled to the individual need [29]. Our preferred method to address long bone non-union in the lower extremity differs depending on the non-union type to be revised [2]. In clinically non-infected cases indicated for surgery, our preferred method in the tibial shaft non-union is exchange nailing, where we aim to increase the nail diameter by at least 2 mm and emphasize a good reaming technique, with stepwise reamer increase by 0.5 mm and final reaming at least 1 mm greater than the aspired nail diameter. In the femur, especially in oligotrophic cases, again exchange nailing is our preferred method. In hypertrophic non-unions, especially in the diametaphyseal region, augmentative plating with local cancellous autograft can be a viable option. The simulation presented in this study can help assess the pathogenesis of a non-union, assisting in clinical decision making. Depending on rotational and axial alignment, as well as potential bone defects, our revision strategy is adapted as individually required [2].

As the simulation workflow is already reasonably fast and could increase in precision and speed pending further adaptations, its application in the future could also be seen as a screening tool, providing added socioeconomic effects on top of the decreased patient burden of disease [2]. As it is run on available clinical information alone, it could potentially also be applied centrally through health or accident insurance organizations, allowing for a large number of patients screened early on.

Limitations

This study has several underlying limitations. The introduced simulation protocol and the conclusions drawn are based on the case series analysis of two patients, which limits the generalizability of the results due to the low patient number. The presented study serves only as a description of two use cases of the workflow's clinical applicability. The workflow has been clinically tested in different upper and lower extremity fracture entities during a regular healing course, showing its principal accuracy in union determination [24,25]. In contrast, the current analysis was performed to show its clinical application in challenging healing cases with complex fractures and patients with different pre-existing diseases representing the influence of both mechanical and biological factors on fracture healing, leading to non-union. The determined effects on tissue differentiation cannot be validated experimentally in vivo. Validation can only be given through the observed clinical course in line with the simulation results. The mechanical parameters that the simulation is based on are determined by the implant and weight-bearing condition assumed as per the patient's body weight. More detailed simulations incorporate musculoskeletal models including muscle and tendon pull based on individualized motion capture to provide a greater degree of detail and with higher resolution in the fracture gap [21]. CT and conventional 2D imaging data were manually matched and aligned, thus introducing potential bias. Another limitation to be mentioned is the possible alterations in gait and weight-bearing after a lower limb fracture. It has to be assumed that patients reduce their weight-bearing when suffering pain. As our second case shows, this has to be taken into consideration in further development and usage of the simulation. However, the combined consideration of both biological and mechanical aspects in the workflow presented here seems to make up for this detail, still providing a simulation result according to the clinical course.

It can be expected that in the future, by incorporating additional clinical data types in more diverse study setups, also including different and more complex fractures and varying patient conditions, the precision of the model's predictive capability will certainly increase [37–40]. This could potentially lead to adapted treatment, as well as aftercare regimes, such as addressing weight-bearing according to the fracture needs [41,42].

5. Conclusions

We introduce a workflow that may improve success in predicting fractures at risk for non-union development early during the treatment course in a clinical application scenario. In this use case series, for each patient, the input necessary for simulation is based on available clinical and radiographic information. Further validation in a large non-union cohort is needed to increase the model's precision, especially in biologically challenging cases, and show its validity as a screening instrument compared to established clinical scores.

Supplementary Materials: The following supporting information can be downloaded at: https://www.mdpi.com/article/10.3390/jcm13133922/s1, Figure S1: Modeled mechanobiological processes of the Ulm tissue-level bone healing model; Figure S2: Steps to apply the simulation model to the investigated cases; Figure S3: Segmentation of the CT data in 3D slicer. Yellow: Bone; Blue: Nail Implant; Violett: Fibula Implant; Figure S4 Meshed investigate femur case with the mentioned healing domain. Depicted in a sliced view from AP; Figure S5 Applied loading condition in the femur case; Figure S6 User interface to track simulation status and analyze the simulation results, provided by OSORA medical GmbH.

Author Contributions: Methodology: F.N. and L.E.; data curation: B.J.B., F.N., L.E., Y.S., T.C.M. and M.M.M.; visualization: T.C.M., F.N. and Y.S.; writing—original draft preparation: T.C.M., S.L. and B.J.B.; writing—review and editing: F.E., S.L., L.E., F.N., T.H., M.M.M. and M.K.R.; conceptualization: B.J.B., F.E., F.N. and L.E.; supervision: B.J.B. and T.H.; project administration: B.J.B. All authors have read and agreed to the published version of the manuscript.

Funding: Exist Research Grand: 03EFQBW222.

Institutional Review Board Statement: Ethical approval was obtained from the ethical committee of Tuebingen University (application number 318/2022BO2, 840/2019B02; approval date 13 July 2022).

Informed Consent Statement: Informed consent was given by both patients to participate in the collection of movement data and the fracture and non-union simulation based on their clinical and imaging data, as well as their publication. Additional consent was given to share the data with the simulation provider.

Data Availability Statement: Data supporting this study beyond the presented information are not available.

Conflicts of Interest: The authors declare that this research was conducted in the absence of any commercial or financial relationships that could be construed as a potential conflict of interest.

References

1. Zura, R.; Xiong, Z.; Einhorn, T.; Watson, J.T.; Ostrum, R.F.; Prayson, M.J.; Della Rocca, G.J.; Mehta, S.; McKinley, T.; Wang, Z.; et al. Epidemiology of Fracture Nonunion in 18 Human Bones. *JAMA Surg.* **2016**, *151*, e162775. [CrossRef] [PubMed]
2. Braun, B.J.; Menger, M.M.; Reumann, M.K.; Histing, T. Pseudarthrosen beim Erwachsenen—Ein Update. *Orthopädie Und Unfallchirurgie Up2date* **2022**, *17*, 537–558. [CrossRef]
3. Nicholson, J.A.; Makaram, N.; Simpson, A.; Keating, J.F. Fracture nonunion in long bones: A literature review of risk factors and surgical management. *Injury* **2021**, *52*, S3–S11. [CrossRef] [PubMed]
4. Lynch, J.R.; Taitsman, L.A.; Barei, D.P.; Nork, S.E. Femoral nonunion: Risk factors and treatment options. *J. Am. Acad. Orthop. Surg.* **2008**, *16*, 88–97. [CrossRef] [PubMed]
5. Copuroglu, C.; Calori, G.M.; Giannoudis, P.V. Fracture non-union: Who is at risk? *Injury* **2013**, *44*, 1379–1382. [CrossRef] [PubMed]
6. Santolini, E.; West, R.; Giannoudis, P.V. Risk factors for long bone fracture non-union: A stratification approach based on the level of the existing scientific evidence. *Injury* **2015**, *46*, S8–S19. [CrossRef]
7. Brinker, M.R.; Hanus, B.D.; Sen, M.; O'Connor, D.P. The devastating effects of tibial nonunion on health-related quality of life. *J. Bone Joint Surg. Am.* **2013**, *95*, 2170–2176. [CrossRef] [PubMed]

8. Rupp, M.; Biehl, C.; Budak, M.; Thormann, U.; Heiss, C.; Alt, V. Diaphyseal long bone nonunions—Types, aetiology, economics, and treatment recommendations. *Int. Orthop.* **2018**, *42*, 247–258. [CrossRef] [PubMed]
9. Hak, D.J.; Fitzpatrick, D.; Bishop, J.A.; Marsh, J.L.; Tilp, S.; Schnettler, R.; Simpson, H.; Alt, V. Delayed union and nonunions: Epidemiology, clinical issues, and financial aspects. *Injury* **2014**, *45*, S3–S7. [CrossRef]
10. Bhandari, M.; Guyatt, G.H.; Swiontkowski, M.F.; Tornetta, P., 3rd; Sprague, S.; Schemitsch, E.H. A lack of consensus in the assessment of fracture healing among orthopaedic surgeons. *J. Orthop. Trauma* **2002**, *16*, 562–566. [CrossRef]
11. Ferreira, N.; Marais, L.; Aldous, C. Challenges and controversies in defining and classifying tibial non-unions. *SA Orthop. J.* **2014**, *13*, 52–56.
12. Wittauer, M.; Burch, M.A.; McNally, M.; Vandendriessche, T.; Clauss, M.; Della Rocca, G.J.; Giannoudis, P.V.; Metsemakers, W.J.; Morgenstern, M. Definition of long-bone nonunion: A scoping review of prospective clinical trials to evaluate current practice. *Injury* **2021**, *52*, 3200–3205. [CrossRef]
13. Neumaier, M.; Biberthaler, P. Hypertrophe Pseudarthrose. In *Knochendefekte und Pseudarthrosen*; Biberthaler, P., van Griensven, M., Eds.; Springer: Berlin, Heidelberg, 2017; pp. 77–100. [CrossRef]
14. Schmidmaier, G. Non Unions. *Unfallchirurg* **2020**, *123*, 669–670. [CrossRef]
15. Simpson, A. The forgotten phase of fracture healing: The need to predict nonunion. *Bone Joint Res.* **2017**, *6*, 610–611. [CrossRef]
16. Claes, L. Biomechanical Principles and Mechanobiologic Aspects of Flexible and Locked Plating. *J. Orthop. Trauma* **2011**, *25*, S4–S7. [CrossRef]
17. Claes, L. Mechanobiology of fracture healing part 1: Principles. *Unfallchirurg* **2017**, *120*, 14–22. [CrossRef]
18. Gerstenfeld, L.C.; Cullinane, D.M.; Barnes, G.L.; Graves, D.T.; Einhorn, T.A. Fracture healing as a post-natal developmental process: Molecular, spatial, and temporal aspects of its regulation. *J. Cell Biochem.* **2003**, *88*, 873–884. [CrossRef]
19. Einhorn, T.A.; Gerstenfeld, L.C. Fracture healing: Mechanisms and interventions. *Nat. Rev. Rheumatol.* **2015**, *11*, 45–54. [CrossRef]
20. Marmor, M.T.; Dailey, H.; Marcucio, R.; Hunt, A.C. Biomedical research models in the science of fracture healing—Pitfalls & promises. *Injury* **2020**, *51*, 2118–2128. [CrossRef]
21. Braun, B.J.; Orth, M.; Diebels, S.; Wickert, K.; Andres, A.; Gawlitza, J.; Bücker, A.; Pohlemann, T.; Roland, M. Individualized Determination of the Mechanical Fracture Environment After Tibial Exchange Nailing-A Simulation-Based Feasibility Study. *Front. Surg.* **2021**, *8*, 749209. [CrossRef]
22. Orth, M.; Ganse, B.; Andres, A.; Wickert, K.; Warmerdam, E.; Müller, M.; Diebels, S.; Roland, M.; Pohlemann, T. Simulation-based prediction of bone healing and treatment recommendations for lower leg fractures: Effects of motion, weight-bearing and fibular mechanics. *Front. Bioeng. Biotechnol.* **2023**, *11*, 1067845. [CrossRef]
23. Niemeyer, F.; Claes, L.; Ignatius, A.; Meyers, N.; Simon, U. Simulating lateral distraction osteogenesis. *PLoS ONE* **2018**, *13*, e0194500. [CrossRef]
24. Engelhardt, L.; Niemeyer, F.; Christen, P.; Müller, R.; Stock, K.; Blauth, M.; Urban, K.; Ignatius, A.; Simon, U. Simulating Metaphyseal Fracture Healing in the Distal Radius. *Biomechanics* **2021**, *1*, 29–42. [CrossRef]
25. Degenhart, C.; Engelhardt, L.; Niemeyer, F.; Erne, F.; Braun, B.; Gebhard, F.; Schütze, K. Computer-Based Mechanobiological Fracture Healing Model Predicts Non-Union of Surgically Treated Diaphyseal Femur Fractures. *J. Clin. Med.* **2023**, *12*, 3461. [CrossRef]
26. Simon, U.; Augat, P.; Utz, M.; Claes, L. A numerical model of the fracture healing process that describes tissue development and revascularisation. *Comput. Methods Biomech. Biomed. Eng.* **2011**, *14*, 79–93. [CrossRef]
27. Pauwels, F. Eine neue Theorie über den Einfluß mechanischer Reize auf die Differenzierung der Stützgewebe. *Z. Anat. Entwicklungsgeschichte* **1960**, *121*, 478–515. [CrossRef]
28. Claes, L.E.; Heigele, C.A. Magnitudes of local stress and strain along bony surfaces predict the course and type of fracture healing. *J. Biomech.* **1999**, *32*, 255–266. [CrossRef]
29. Fedorov, A.; Beichel, R.; Kalpathy-Cramer, J.; Finet, J.; Fillion-Robin, J.C.; Pujol, S.; Bauer, C.; Jennings, D.; Fennessy, F.; Sonka, M.; et al. 3D Slicer as an image computing platform for the Quantitative Imaging Network. *Magn. Reson. Imaging* **2012**, *30*, 1323–1341. [CrossRef]
30. Heller, M.O.; Bergmann, G.; Kassi, J.P.; Claes, L.; Haas, N.P.; Duda, G.N. Determination of muscle loading at the hip joint for use in pre-clinical testing. *J. Biomech.* **2005**, *38*, 1155–1163. [CrossRef]
31. Zhao, D.; Banks, S.A.; D'Lima, D.D.; Colwell, C.W., Jr.; Fregly, B.J. In vivo medial and lateral tibial loads during dynamic and high flexion activities. *J. Orthop. Res.* **2007**, *25*, 593–602. [CrossRef]
32. O'Halloran, K.; Coale, M.; Costales, T.; Zerhusen, T., Jr.; Castillo, R.C.; Nascone, J.W.; O'Toole, R.V. Will My Tibial Fracture Heal? Predicting Nonunion at the Time of Definitive Fixation Based on Commonly Available Variables. *Clin. Orthop. Relat. Res.* **2016**, *474*, 1385–1395. [CrossRef]
33. Chloros, G.D.; Kanakaris, N.K.; Vun, J.S.H.; Howard, A.; Giannoudis, P.V. Scoring systems for early prediction of tibial fracture non-union: An update. *Int. Orthop.* **2021**, *45*, 2081–2091. [CrossRef]
34. Chloros, G.D.; Howard, A.; Giordano, V.; Giannoudis, P.V. Radiographic Long Bone Fracture Healing Scores: Can they predict non-union? *Injury* **2020**, *51*, 1693–1695. [CrossRef]
35. Dailey, H.L.; Schwarzenberg, P.; Daly, C.J.; Boran, S.A.M.; Maher, M.M.; Harty, J.A. Virtual Mechanical Testing Based on Low-Dose Computed Tomography Scans for Tibial Fracture: A Pilot Study of Prediction of Time to Union and Comparison with Subjective Outcomes Scoring. *J. Bone Joint. Surg. Am.* **2019**, *101*, 1193–1202. [CrossRef]

36. Millar, M.J.; Wilkinson, A.; Navarre, P.; Steiner, J.; Vohora, A.; Hardidge, A.; Edwards, E. Nail Fit: Does Nail Diameter to Canal Ratio Predict the Need for Exchange Nailing in the Setting of Aseptic, Hypertrophic Femoral Nonunions? *J. Orthop. Trauma* **2018**, *32*, 245–250. [CrossRef]
37. Ghiasi, M.S.; Chen, J.; Vaziri, A.; Rodriguez, E.K.; Nazarian, A. Bone fracture healing in mechanobiological modeling: A review of principles and methods. *Bone Rep.* **2017**, *6*, 87–100. [CrossRef]
38. Ghiasi, M.S.; Chen, J.E.; Rodriguez, E.K.; Vaziri, A.; Nazarian, A. Computational modeling of human bone fracture healing affected by different conditions of initial healing stage. *BMC Musculoskelet. Disord.* **2019**, *20*, 562. [CrossRef]
39. Wang, M.; Yang, N.; Wang, X. A review of computational models of bone fracture healing. *Med. Biol. Eng. Comput.* **2017**, *55*, 1895–1914. [CrossRef]
40. Claes, L. Improvement of clinical fracture healing—What can be learned from mechano-biological research? *J. Biomech.* **2021**, *115*, 110148. [CrossRef]
41. Glatt, V.; Evans, C.H.; Tetsworth, K. A Concert between Biology and Biomechanics: The Influence of the Mechanical Environment on Bone Healing. *Front Physiol.* **2016**, *7*, 678. [CrossRef]
42. Hart, N.H.; Nimphius, S.; Rantalainen, T.; Ireland, A.; Siafarikas, A.; Newton, R.U. Mechanical basis of bone strength: Influence of bone material, bone structure and muscle action. *J. Musculoskelet. Neuronal Interact.* **2017**, *17*, 114–139. [PubMed]

Journal of
Clinical Medicine

MDPI

Article

Pediatric Diaphyseal Forearm Fracture Management with Biodegradable Poly-L-Lactide-Co-Glycolide (PLGA) Intramedullary Implants: A Longitudinal Study

Aba Lőrincz [1,2,3], Ágnes Mária Lengyel [3], András Kedves [2], Hermann Nudelman [1,3] and Gergő Józsa [1,3,*]

1 Department of Thermophysiology, Institute for Translational Medicine, Medical School, University of Pécs, 12 Szigeti Street, 7624 Pécs, Hungary; aba.lorincz@gmail.com (A.L.); nuhwaao.pte@tr.pte.hu (H.N.)
2 Institute of Information and Electrical Technology, Faculty of Engineering and Information Technology, University of Pécs, Boszorkány Street 2, 7624 Pécs, Hungary; kedvesandras94@gmail.com
3 Division of Pediatric Surgery, Traumatology, Urology and Pediatric Otolaryngology, Department of Pediatrics, Clinical Complex, University of Pécs, 7 József Attila Street, 7623 Pécs, Hungary; suzd1j@pte.hu
* Correspondence: jozsa.gergo@pte.hu; Tel.: +36-30-514-2730

Abstract: Background: Pediatric forearm fractures represent a substantial proportion of childhood injuries, requiring effective and minimally invasive treatments. Our study investigated the mid-term outcomes of biodegradable poly-L-lactide-co-glycolide (PLGA) intramedullary implants in managing diaphyseal forearm fractures in children. **Methods:** A follow-up cohort study was conducted with 38 patients treated with PLGA implants. Control examinations were performed one year post-operation, assessing bone healing through radiographic evaluations and functional outcomes using injured and uninjured limb range of motion (ROM) comparisons. Scarring was evaluated employing the Vancouver Scar Scale (VSS), and satisfaction via a questionnaire. **Results:** Children were predominantly female (76.4%), with a mean age of 9.71 (SD: 2.69) years. Effective fracture stabilization and bone healing were found in all patients, with a minor reduction (mean difference of −1.5°, $p = 0.282$) in elbow flexion on the operated side (139.3°) compared to the intact (140.8°). Elbow extension presented negligible average changes (0.2°, $p = 0.098$). Forearm movements were slightly reduced on the operated side (mean pronation: 80.8° vs. 83.7°, $p = 0.166$; average supination: 83.5° vs. 85.7°, $p = 0.141$). Wrist palmar flexion and dorsiflexion showed no significant differences. VSS ratings indicated minimal scarring (mean guardian and doctor scores were 1.13 and 0.55, respectively, $p = 0.020$), and all patients reported satisfaction with the treatment outcomes. **Conclusions:** Biodegradable implants are effective for pediatric forearm fractures, providing stable bone healing while preserving functional ROM with minimal scarring and high patient satisfaction. PLGA proved to be a viable alternative to traditional metal implants, eliminating secondary removal surgeries.

Keywords: pediatric; diaphyseal; forearm; fracture; biodegradable; implants; intramedullary; poly-L-lactide-co-glycolide (PLGA); follow-up

1. Introduction

Among pediatric skeletal injuries, forearm fractures represent a prevalent and clinically significant challenge, accounting for approximately 17.8% of all childhood fractures in the United States, out of an annual incidence rate of 9.47 per 1000 children [1]. The later this damage is adequately addressed, the more severe the resultant loss of forearm motion and subsequent functional and social limitations in performing the activities of daily living, along with the psychological and esthetic impact [2]. The anatomy of the pediatric forearm provides essential guidance for fracture management. Relatively, the ulna is straight and static, while the radius is curved and rotates over the ulna during pronation and supination [3]. These bones are connected by the interosseous membrane in the middle and at the joints—both at the wrist and elbow through the proximal and distal radioulnar joints.

Each bone has a proximal and distal physis, with the distal physis contributing significantly to longitudinal growth, accounting for 75% in the radius and 81% in the ulna [4]. Growth polarization correlates with observations that fractures nearer to the distal ends have a higher remodeling potential than those closer to the elbow.

Location and nature of the fracture change with age; complete, displaced fractures are more common in adolescence, while younger children more frequently experience plastic deformation or greenstick fractures [5]. Bilateral forearm fractures often result from indirect trauma, most commonly from falling onto an outstretched hand (FOOSH) [2]. During a fall, a child typically extends the arm to protect against the impact, stiffening the wrist, which leads to fracture due to the axial load that can injure the hand, wrist, forearm, elbow, and shoulder.

Deformities of the limb can indicate a FOOSH injury, but the diagnosis is primarily confirmed through anteroposterior (AP) and lateral orthogonal forearm radiographs, occasionally supplemented by CT or MR scans [6]. Alternatively, a recent trial found the cost-effective, rapid, and radiation-free ultrasound to be a viable diagnostic option [7]. Distal pulses and capillary refill must be assessed too. Direct impacts can also cause isolated ulnar mid-shaft fractures ("nightstick fractures") or, less commonly, of the radius. Abuse should be considered in children younger than three years old [8].

Classification of pediatric diaphyseal fractures can be performed using the internationally employed "AO Pediatric Comprehensive Classification of Long-Bone Fractures" (PCCF), which provides detailed guidelines for categorizing fractures based on the location and morphology of the break and covering different segments and subsegments of long bones [9]. Fracture location is designated by numbers: the forearm bones are labeled as "2", the proximal segment as "1", the diaphyseal as "2", and the distal as "3". The letters "r" and "u" denote the radius and ulna, respectively. The specific subsegment of the bone (epiphysis, metaphysis, diaphysis) is indicated by "E", "M", and "D". The second part of the code describes fracture morphology, including patterns specific to children. Severity is separated by a dot (.) and classified into two levels: simple (1) and comminuted (broken into multiple fragments) (2). Displacement is indicated by Roman numerals aiding in a clear and concise description of fractures. In cases where the fracture involves the growth plate, the Salter and Harris classification is utilized [10].

Conservative therapy, which primarily involves immobilization with a cast, is a widely accepted and effective treatment for pediatric forearm fractures, especially when displacement is minimal [8]. Typically, conservative treatment includes closed reduction followed by casting to restore alignment and immobilize the fracture. Casting type and duration depend on the characteristics of the fracture and the age of the child; for example, children under ten with angulations less than ten degrees often achieve complete remodeling and good function with casting alone. Intact periosteum in many of these fractures enhances stability and facilitates natural splinting, making conservative treatment particularly effective. For greenstick fractures, this is especially true, where the bone bends and cracks without breaking completely [11]. Younger children benefit significantly from this method due to the higher remodeling potential of their bones, allowing for healing with minimal intervention and good functional outcomes. However, careful monitoring is essential to prevent complications such as repeated displacement, inadequate healing, or joint stiffness, with follow-up X-rays ensuring proper alignment. Despite these challenges, conservative therapy remains a cornerstone of pediatric fracture management, offering a less invasive option with excellent outcomes in many cases.

Operative therapy serves as a critical intervention for pediatric forearm fractures that are unstable, significantly displaced, involving both the radius and ulna, or unresponsive to conservative treatment [12]. Warranting proper alignment and stability is essential for optimal healing and function preventing long-term complications.

Elastic stable intramedullary nailing (ESIN) is a widely employed minimally invasive procedure for pediatric forearm fractures, which involves inserting flexible, strong metal rods into the medullary cavity of the bone, providing internal stabilization [13,14]. Advantages of ESIN include small incisions, reduced postoperative pain, and fast recovery times while allowing early mobilization, beneficial for maintaining muscle strength and joint function compared to metal plating [12]. Due to some drawbacks of metal implants, new resorbable intramedullary implants have been developed for the surgical treatment of pediatric forearm diaphyseal fractures, composed of biodegradable materials such as poly-L-lactide-co-glycolide (PLGA). They offer temporary support during the healing process while gradually dissolving within the body, eliminating the need for a secondary procedure to remove the hardware and all associated complications [15].

Surgical intervention carries inherent risks, such as nerve injury, infection, or anesthesia-related respiratory depression, but the benefits often outweigh these concerns in appropriately selected cases. Ensuring accurate bone healing, restoring full function, and preventing long-term sequelae such as deformity or chronic pain remain the primary objectives of operative therapy. Therefore, PLGA implants seem particularly advantageous for fractures of the radius, ulna, or both, provided proper immobilization is ensured [16,17]. However, they may not be suitable for oblique spiral, comminuted, or epiphyseal fractures, and are contraindicated in the presence of local infection or poor patient compliance [16].

For complex fractures, plate and screw fixation is often employed to ensure precise alignment of the fracture. This intervention proves particularly effective for fractures near joints or those that are comminuted, providing robust stability and promoting proper healing [8]. External fixation (fixateur externe) is another valuable option involving the stabilization of the bones from outside the body using a frame attached with pins or wires, allowing for adjustment, and it is particularly useful in managing complex fractures with extensive soft tissue injuries [18]. Hybrid fixation combines different methods to achieve optimal results [19].

Despite the apparent advantages of resorbable implants, research on their use in pediatric populations has been limited. Only two studies have investigated the outcomes of intramedullary PLGA implants for pediatric diaphyseal forearm fractures for an extended period, with follow-ups at two [20] and four [17] years post-surgery. Another trial focused on distal fracture management [21]. Therefore, our study aims to assess the mid-term functional and cosmetic results of bioabsorbable intramedullary implants in treating this common condition, providing a deeper understanding of their capabilities in pediatric diaphyseal forearm fractures.

2. Materials and Methods

2.1. Study Design and Patient Selection

A single-center, single-arm, descriptive cohort follow-up study was conducted at the Pediatric Surgical Division of the University of Pécs in accordance with the Strengthening the Reporting of Observational Studies in Epidemiology (STROBE) guidelines [22]. Data were retrospectively collected from our hospital's recordings of pediatric patients who consecutively underwent surgery for diaphyseal forearm fractures using PLGA intramedullary implants between May 2021 and March 2023. Then, they were prospectively recalled to evaluate their functional, esthetic, and psychological recovery one year post-surgery.

A total of 38 pediatric patients met the inclusion criteria, which were (1) pediatric patients under the age of 18 years at the time of follow-up with (2) forearm fractures treated with absorbable intramedullary PLGA implants, (3) the time between injury and surgery was within eight days, and (4) they had at least one year of postoperative recovery. Eight patients were excluded due to loss of follow-up attributable to (1) missing contact information, (2) not appearing for control examination, (3) or because of bilateral fractures. Children with (4) oblique spiral, (5) multi-fragmented, or (6) epiphyseal fractures, (7) presence of local infection, (8) poor compliance, and (9) bone remodeling affecting comorbidity or (10) medication would have been also excluded; however, no patient was admitted with these conditions during the investigation period.

2.2. Intervention

PLGA implants (Activa IM-Nail™, Bioretec Ltd., Tampere, Finland) function by maintaining their mechanical strength throughout the critical period of bone healing (Figure 1).

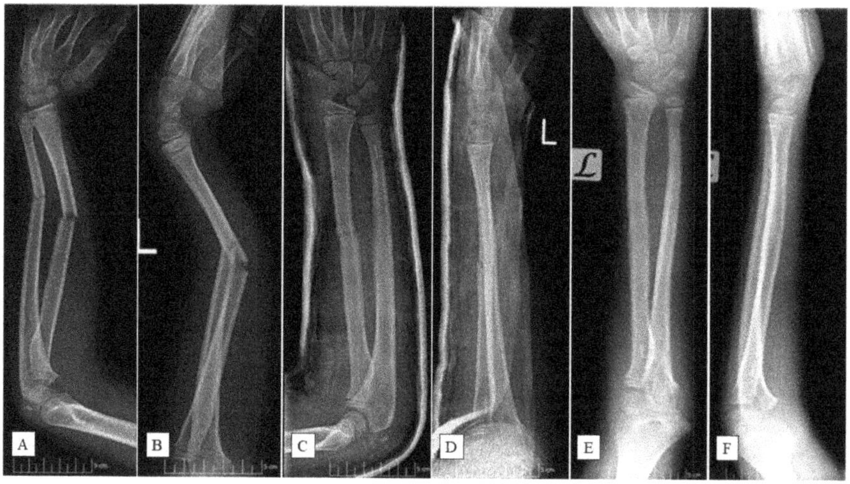

Figure 1. An 11-year-old boy fell while playing football and had a deformed left (L) arm. Preoperative anteroposterior (AP) (**A**) and lateral (**B**) radiographic views of the forearm exposed subperiosteal fractures of both ulna and radius. X-rays post-surgery ((**C**)—AP, (**D**)—lateral aspects) show the successful insertion of PLGA implants, confirmed by the radiopaque markers. Six-month control images ((**E**)—AP, (**F**)—lateral views) revealed completely healed fractures with good axial alignment.

These polymers degrade through hydrolysis, breaking down into lactic acid and glycolic acid monomers [23,24]. Subsequently, the monomers are metabolized via the citric acid cycle, producing water and carbon dioxide as end products. This process lowers the local pH, creating an acidic environment around the implant which facilitates its gradual resorption. Complete degradation of PLGA typically occurs within 9–12 months, making it a reliable material for temporary internal fixation in pediatric patients [25]. Additionally, the implants feature a tricalcium phosphate (β-TCP) marker for precise fluoroscopic placement (Figure 1C–F).

2.3. Surgical Protocol

Several key steps are involved in the surgical procedure for inserting PLGA implants in a minimally invasive manner. After cleaning and disinfecting the operative area and administering general anesthesia, the patient was positioned supine with the affected arm placed on a radiolucent table. Additional management, such as analgesia with 0.1–0.2 mg/kg nalbuphine injections (Nubain, ALTAMEDICS GmbH, Cologne, Germany), and sedation with midazolam (Dormicum, Egis Gyógyszergyár Zrt, Budapest, Hungary), were administered perioperatively based on clinical indications and parental consent. Small incisions were made dorsally on the distal radius and laterally on the proximal ulna. Entry points into the cortical bone had been created using an awl or drill. For the radius, an entry hole was made by positioning the drill perpendicular to the cortex and gradually angling it to form the smallest possible angle with the diaphyseal axis. Then, the medullary canal was reamed with a dilator that matched the implant size—and this process was repeated for the ulna. Implant diameter choice is critical and should match the smallest diameter of the medullary canal, with available options being 2.7 and 3.2 mm in diameter, and lengths of 200, 300, and 400 mm.

Once the canals were prepared, the PLGA implants were introduced using an inserter, guaranteeing no rotational movements to prevent misalignment. Fluoroscopy was used to verify implant positions, with the β-TCP tips aiding in visualization. Protruding ends of the implants were trimmed and smoothed to avoid soft tissue irritation, and the incisions were closed with absorbable sutures. Postoperative care includes immobilizing the limb in a cast above the elbow at a 90-degree angle for 4–6 weeks, with sports and strenuous activities avoided for 2–6 months.

2.4. Evaluated Metrics

Endpoints included patient demographics (such as age, sex, dominant hand) and fracture characteristics (time of injury, and affected side and bone), collected in Microsoft Excel 2021 (Microsoft Corporation, Redmond, WA, USA). Primary outcomes included the joint function evaluation one year after surgery via their range of motion (ROM) using a goniometer. ROM was calculated by adding the absolute values of opposing motions. Measurements from the operated extremity were compared to those of the unharmed limb to determine any discrepancies in ROM for the following movements:

- Elbow flexion and extension: Normal range is −10 to 150 degrees (°). Patients were instructed to fully extend and flex their elbows while standing with arms at their sides (Figure 2).
- Forearm pronation and supination: The standard interval is 80 to 90° in both directions from the neutral position. Children held a pen in a fist with elbows at 90°, rotating their forearms to achieve maximum pronation and supination (Figure 3A,B).
- Wrist palmar flexion and dorsiflexion: Typical ROM is 80° dorsiflexion and 70° palmar flexion. Patients placed their forearms on a horizontal surface, moving their wrists to the maximum palmar and dorsiflexion positions (Figure 3C–F).

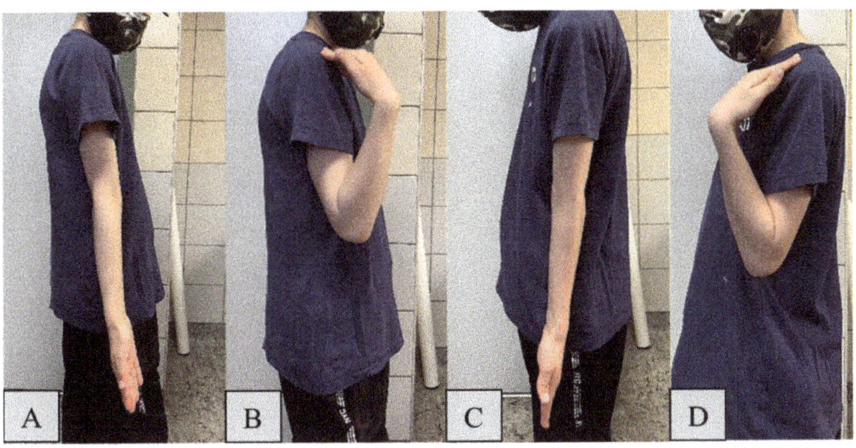

Figure 2. Elbow extension (**A**) and flexion (**B**) of the uninjured arm of an 11-year-old boy. One year after surgery, the operated arm's cubital extension (**C**) and flexion (**D**) demonstrate intact functionality.

X-rays were employed to assess the remodeling of the bones (Figure 4A,B), while surgical scars were evaluated using the Vancouver Scar Scale (VSS) (Figure 4C,D) [26], calculating the composite score of four criteria:

- Pigmentation: scored from 0 (normal) to 2 (severe hyperpigmentation).
- Vascularity: counted from 0 (normal) to 3 (severe vascularity).
- Pliability: graded from 0 (normal) to 5 (severe contracture).
- Height: recorded from 0 (flat) to 3 (more than 5 mm).

Satisfaction was assessed through a questionnaire asking if the patient or their guardian would choose the same surgical method again under similar circumstances. This survey aimed to capture subjective satisfaction with the functional and aesthetic outcomes of the surgery.

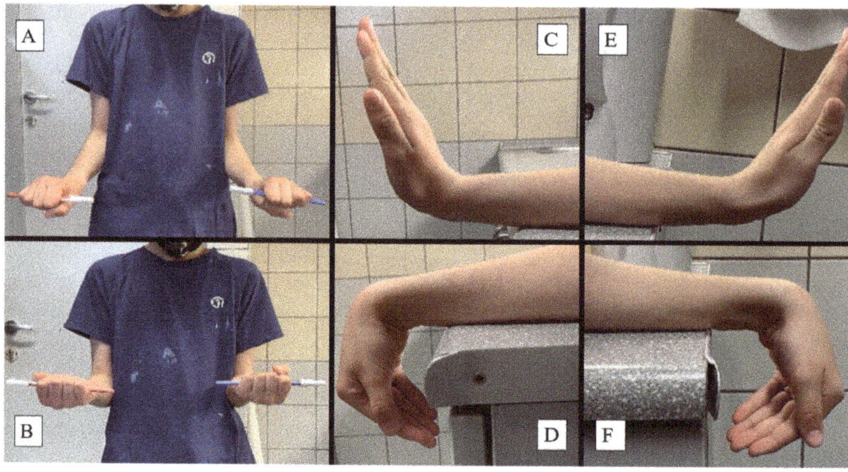

Figure 3. One year post-PLGA implantation: Images showing the pronation (**A**) and supination (**B**) of the forearm, while the intact hand holds a red pen and the healed grasps the blue writing implement. Baseline wrist function is demonstrated with the dorsal (**C**) and palmar flexion (**D**) of the uninjured extremity, which can be compared to the ROM of the operated arm (**E**,**F**).

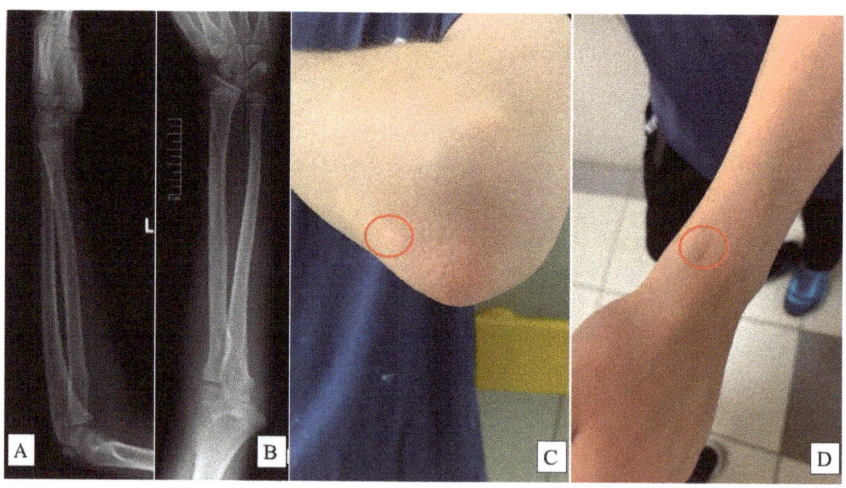

Figure 4. X-rays captured at the one-year follow-up examination of a L pediatric forearm fracture treated with PLGA implants from lateral (**A**) and AP (**B**) views showing intact bone growth and development. Surgical scars—highlighted by the red circles—were evaluated via the Vancouver Scar Scale (VSS) on the olecranon ((**C**), 0 point) and the distal end of the radius ((**D**), 1 point).

2.5. Data Analysis and Visualization

Descriptive statistics were calculated until two decimals for all continuous outcomes utilizing means, standard deviations (SDs), medians, interquartile ranges (IQRs), 25th percentiles (IQR25s), 75th percentiles (IQR75s), counts, and ranges, while discrete endpoints were analyzed via count and percentage distributions. This study employed Python 3.12.3 (Python Software Foundation, Wilmington, DE, USA) for data visualization and statistical analysis, a versatile and open-source language that facilitated data handling and testing operating several specialized libraries. Statistical analysis was conducted using SciPy and NumPy libraries. The Shapiro–Wilk test was utilized to determine normality, suitable for smaller sample sizes. Two-sample *t*-tests were used to compare means from two independent groups when both samples were normally distributed, while nonparametric Mann–Whitney U-tests differentiated not normally distributed samples. Additionally, a chi-square (χ^2) test determined the association between categorical variables. Differences were deemed significant at $p \leq 0.05$. Matplotlib was utilized for fundamental plot creation and customization, while Seaborn provided advanced plotting functions and aesthetic enhancements.

3. Results

This study included 38 pediatric patients with diaphyseal forearm fractures treated using PLGA implants. Patients age ranged from 5 to 15 years, with a mean age of 9.71 (SD = 2.69) years. Regarding sex distribution, the majority of the patients (76.32% of all cases) were female, and the affected side was more often the right forearm (55.26%, $n = 21$) (Table 1). Dominant hand analysis revealed that 85.71% ($n = 18$) of the patients were right-handed; moreover, the nondominant hand was involved in slightly more (52.12%, $n = 12$) injuries, which was not statistically significant ($p = 0.513$). In terms of fracture type, most of the fractures involved both the radius and ulna (84.21%, $n = 32$), with only five children (13.16%) having fractures of the radius alone and one patient (2.63%) having a fracture of the ulna alone. Restricted elbow flexion (<137°) was linked significantly ($p = 0.017$) with radius-only fractures (80% of patients had limited mobility), while wide ROM (≥137°) was marginally associated ($p = 0.052$) with fractures of both bones (64.52% of children had high mobility).

Table 1. Discrete outcome distribution of children and their PLGA-treated diaphyseal forearm fractures, one year post-operation.

Variable	Category	Count	Percentage
Sex	Female	29	76.32%
	Male	9	23.68%
Affected side	Left	17	44.74%
	Right	21	55.26%
Fracture type	Radius	5	13.16%
	Both	32	84.21%
	Ulna	1	2.63%
Dominant hand	Right	18	85.71%
	Left	3	14.29%
Satisfaction	Satisfied	38	100.00%

Functional outcomes were assessed via ROM for various movements of the forearm, including the elbow and wrist performance as well, and are summarized in Table 2 and visualized in Figure 5.

For elbow flexion, the mean maximum angle for the operated side was 139.3° (SD = 6.2), compared to 140.8° (SD = 6.2) on the intact side. The minor reduction of −1.45° on the operated side suggests effective restoration of function by the PLGA implants, despite a statistically significant difference ($p = 0.282$). Elbow extension showed mean ROM values of −1.1° (SD = 2.9) for the PLGA-treated and −1.3° (SD = 2.9) for the intact side, with a negligible mean difference of 0.05° ($p = 0.098$), indicating that the surgical intervention had no significant impact on extension capability.

Forearm pronation exhibited a mean ROM of 80.8° (SD = 6.6) on the operated side and 82.4° (SD = 6.6) on the intact side. The slight reduction of −1.61° in pronation on the operated side ($p = 0.166$), suggests a clinically minimal impact on rotational movement. Supination of the forearm demonstrated a mean ROM loss of 0.24° ($p = 0.141$) for the operated side, representing no significant difference and, thus, supporting the efficacy of the PLGA implants in maintaining rotational movement.

Table 2. Descriptive statistics of continuous variables from 38 PLGA-treated, diaphyseal forearm fractured children, based on data collected during one-year follow-up examinations.

Endpoint (Unit)	Region	Status	Mean	SD	Min	Max	Median	IQR	IQR25	IQR75
Age (years)	∞	Child	9.71	2.69	5.00	15.00	10.00	4.00	8.00	12.00
Flexion (°)	Elbow	Operated	139.30	6.20	130.00	155.00	140.50	8.25	136.50	144.75
		Intact	140.80	6.20	130.00	155.00	140.50	8.25	136.50	144.75
Extension (°)		Operated	−1.10	2.90	−10.00	0.00	0.00	3.00	−3.00	0.00
		Intact	−1.30	2.90	−10.00	0.00	0.00	3.00	−3.00	0.00
Pronation (°)	Forearm	Operated	80.80	6.60	70.00	90.00	85.00	6.75	83.25	90.00
		Intact	83.70	6.60	75.00	90.00	85.00	6.75	83.25	90.00
Supination (°)		Operated	83.50	6.60	72.00	110.00	84.00	5.00	80.00	85.00
		Intact	85.70	6.60	75.00	90.00	85.00	6.75	83.25	90.00
Palmar Flexion (°)	Wrist	Operated	64.90	6.70	50.00	75.00	68.00	5.75	65.00	70.75
		Intact	68.60	6.10	50.00	80.00	70.00	7.00	66.50	73.50
Dorsiflexion (°)		Operated	73.20	6.70	60.00	86.00	68.00	6.00	65.00	71.00
		Intact	74.20	6.40	64.00	86.00	72.00	5.00	70.00	75.00
VSS (total score)	Upper Limb	Guardian	1.13	1.14	0.00	4.00	1.00	2.00	0.00	2.00
		Doctor	0.55	0.80	0.00	3.00	0.00	1.00	0.00	1.00

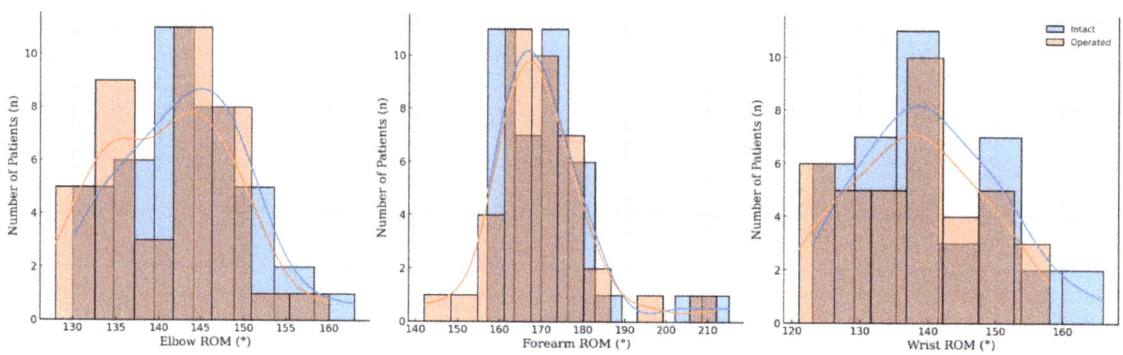

Figure 5. Range of motion (ROM) distributions of pediatric forearm fractured patients one year after PLGA implantation.

Wrist dorsiflexion showed a mean difference of −0.34° (p = 0.070) between the operated and intact sides, representing no significant impact on wrist extension and underscoring the implant's capacity to maintain wrist flexibility. Palmar flexion measurements indicated a mean difference of −0.89° (p = 0.563) between the operated and intact sides, showing no statistically significant variation and highlighting the implant's ability to preserve a wide range of wrist movements.

For the total scores, guardians rated the forearm scars with a mean score of 1.13 (SD = 1.14), while medical professionals provided a significantly (p = 0.020) lower mean VSS score of 0.55 (SD = 0.80). Patient satisfaction was universally high, with all 38 patients reported as satisfied with the treatment outcomes. Comparisons are presented in brief in Table 3.

Table 3. Comparative endpoints one year postoperatively in children with diaphyseal forearm fractures treated with PLGA.

Measurement	Absolute Difference	Relative Difference	Test Used	*p*-Value
Elbow Flexion (°)	−1.45	1.03%	Two-sample t	0.282
Elbow Extension (°)	0.05	3.70%	Two-sample t	0.098
Pronation (°)	−1.61	1.31%	Mann–Whitney U	0.166
Supination (°)	0.24	−3.55%	Mann–Whitney U	0.141
Palmar Flexion (°)	−0.89	1.31%	Two-sample t	0.563
Dorsiflexion (°)	−1.55	−3.55%	Mann–Whitney U	0.070
Dominant Hand Fracture (*n*)	−1	−4.74%	Chi (χ^2)-squared	0.513
VSS (Total Score)	0.58	104.76%	Mann–Whitney U	0.020

4. Discussion

Restoring function while ensuring proper bone healing is the primary objective of pediatric fracture management [8]. Our results indicate that PLGA intramedullary implants are effective in achieving this balance. PLGA is a biodegradable polymer that has garnered attention for its biocompatibility, controlled degradation properties, and minimal toxicity. Due to these characteristics, it is also one of the most promising drug delivery systems in nanoparticle formulation [27]. It is possible to add further active ingredients (such as IGF1) into the implant with timed-release properties, for osteostimulation or to prevent infections [28]. In pediatric traumatology, its features are particularly advantageous, as the implants gradually degrade, eliminating the need for a second surgery to remove hardware [15]. Fewer interventions reduce the overall healthcare burden and mitigate the psychological impact of additional surgical interventions on young patients and their families. Eliminating a second surgical procedure also translates into fewer anesthesia-related risks and a reduced likelihood of peri- and postoperative complications, such as nerve injuries, bleeding, infections, or scar tissue formation, which are particularly pertinent in pediatric populations [29]. Furthermore, the shorter hospital stays and reduced need for follow-up visits significantly decrease the disruption to a child's education and social life, which are vital for their overall development. Despite PLGA materials being generally well tolerated, the potential for allergic reactions or adverse responses in certain patients should be investigated. Additionally, PLGA implants are nearly invisible on X-ray imaging, while they are compatible with MRI. To decrease the cost of control examinations and better compliance, β-TCP bits were incorporated into the tips of the implants, which show up as hyper-opacities on X-ray.

Expanding on our previous investigations [16,30], the current cohort included 38, predominantly female (76.32%), pediatric patients, generally with both of their diaphyses (84.21%) fractured on a single forearm with a mean age of 9.71. A novel observation was that originally, slightly limited elbow flexion (<137°) correlated significantly ($p = 0.017$) with radius-only fractures (80% of patients had restricted mobility), while a broad original ROM (≥137°) was marginally associated ($p = 0.052$) with fractures of both diaphyseal bones (64.52% of children had high mobility)—which might also be significant within a larger analyzed population.

A minor reduction in mean elbow (absolute flexion difference: −1.45°, $p = 0.282$; extension: 0.05°, $p = 0.098$), forearm (pronation: −1.61°, $p = 0.166$; supination: 0.24°, $p = 0.141$), and wrist (palmar flexion: −0.89°, $p = 0.563$; dorsiflexion: −1.55°, $p = 0.070$) mobility highlights the precision of these implants in preserving near-normal ROM. A randomized controlled trial (RCT) found similar patterns regarding preserved ROM using PLGA intramedullary implants [20]. Moreover, they showed that the current gold standard ESIN utilization slightly reduced forearm rotational ROM on the injured side, and increased postoperative pain compared to PLGA intramedullary implants. These findings are significant given the crucial role of elbow and forearm movements in daily activities and play, which are essential for children's development and quality of life. Consistent functional outcomes across ages, genders, and different fracture types underscore the versatility and reliability of PLGA implants.

Another study found that they were also applicable in osteochondral fractures of the lateral condyle of the femur, patella, and radial head [31]. Therefore, the observed uniformity suggests that surgeons can confidently employ these implants across a wide range of fractures, ensuring optimal outcomes irrespective of specific characteristics. This adaptability could be further enhanced by individualizing management to patient needs, considering factors such as the dominant hand and specific activity requirements. Advances in 3D printing and bioengineering could enable the creation of such patient-specific PLGA implants. Tailoring the size and shape of the implants to fit the unique anatomical and physiological needs of each child may improve the effectiveness and comfort of the treatment.

Our results also indicate a generally positive outcome for pediatric forearm fractures treated with PLGA implants, with high satisfaction rates and minor VSS scores, suggesting minimal scarring as assessed by both guardians and doctors. Although both groups gave low total VSS scores, it must be emphasized that guardians rated the scars 104.76% worse than healthcare professionals, which correlates with recent observations [32]. Educating patients and their families about the benefits and care associated with PLGA implants can enhance compliance and satisfaction. Clear communication regarding the implant's degradation process and expected recovery timeline is essential for setting realistic expectations.

Traditional methods of managing pediatric forearm fractures often involve metallic implants, which, while effective, necessitate removal surgeries and pose risks of long-term complications such as hardware irritation or migration [15]. A rigid, nondegradable material may increase postoperative pain and distress, which can lead to a less comfortable recovery period for pediatric patients. Corrosion or mechanical wear can exacerbate cellular toxicity and tissue reactions [33]. Chronic inflammation due to metal debris may also play a role in carcinogenesis [34]. Using PLGA implants circumvents these issues, offering a more patient-friendly approach with fewer long-term risks. Given that PLGA degrades over time, it might also affect the growth plate less [23,24]. A disadvantage of the degradation process is that it is theorized to lead to intermediary byproducts, which are acidic in nature and halt osteoblast activity, thereby hindering recanalization. This has been studied in maxillofacial surgeries and pediatric pelvic osteotomies with over 90% bone recanalization within two years, and another investigation regarding the bone regrowth of the implant canal is underway by Hedelin et al. [35,36]. On the other hand, one of its byproducts, lactate, has a crucial part in biochemical pathways and could exert therapeutic effects such as angiogenesis [37]. Another important consideration is the environmental impact of materials. Metal implants contribute to medical waste and require energy-intensive production processes [38]. In contrast, PLGA implants degrade naturally within the body, reducing the ecological footprint of surgical interventions, and aligning with the broader global efforts toward sustainability in healthcare practices.

Still, there may be cases that require additional stability, such as morbidly obese or hyperactive, noncompliant patients because inadequate fixation can potentially lead to structural rotation, displacement, and shifting. Children with complex, open, pathological, or previous fractures, significant soft-tissue injury, infection in the forearm, metabolic bone or systemic disease, medication affecting bone quality, or fractures older than fourteen days were not yet treated with PLGA and reported in the literature; therefore, careful consideration is necessary [16,17,20]. According to an animal study, resorbable PLGA implants only maintained their maximum stability for eight weeks; thus, if prolonged bone healing or extreme mechanical stress is expected, metallic implants might be more appropriate—albeit they were not analyzed again until the six-month postoperative follow-up, where significant implant resorption was observed [25]. In addition to its accessibility and safe conservation of alignment, ESIN is easier to remove than other operative methods following placement. It also requires shorter periods of hospital admission and anesthesia compared to open approaches [39,40]. ESINs are clearly visible on radiographs and, thus, are easier to manipulate than resorbable implants; however, they are incompatible with magnetic imaging. According to a modified Clavien–Dindo Classification, ESIN was connected to a 9% chance of grade 1 (i.e., asymptomatic delayed union—particularly in children older than 10 years) and 17% of grade 2–4 surgical complications [41]. When using PLGA, there were two implant failures (10.5% of the examined population) [17] and one refracture (1.3%) reported in the literature [16], which were 2.5% (n = 5) for ESIN in both cases [41]. However, we did not encounter these or any complications during the investigation—in addition to the aforementioned slight ROM reductions and minor scars.

Future perspectives and limitations of this research must also be discussed. Expanding the study to include larger and more diverse populations whose data are collected prospectively in a randomized and blinded manner will provide more comprehensive insights into the generalizability of these findings and reduce possible bias. While the current study corroborates the efficacy of PLGA implants in maintaining functional outcomes, future research should explore the long-term effects of these implants on bone health and growth. Given the dynamic nature of pediatric bone development, it is essential to monitor how the gradual degradation of PLGA implants influences bone remodeling over more extended periods. Longitudinal studies tracking patients into adolescence and adulthood would provide valuable insights into any delayed effects and further solidify the implants' safety profile. Additionally, investigating the economic impact of PLGA implants, including cost-effectiveness analyses directly compared to traditional methods, could further substantiate their adoption in clinical practice. Potential research could explore their usefulness in other pediatric traumas, such as fractures of the femur, tibia, or even more complex, multi-fragmentary fractures. Expanding the use of PLGA implants could standardize treatment protocols and streamline surgical training for pediatric surgeons. Lastly, the scar scales and questionnaires are subjective measurements, which could be further objectivized by specialized instruments, such as laser Doppler imaging (LDI) for quantifying scar blood flow, Cutometers for measuring elasticity, or ColorMeters for calculating the melanin index [42]. Using advanced imaging techniques, for example, MRI, would also reveal implant resorption rates [17].

Management of pediatric forearm fractures using PLGA intramedullary implants has demonstrated promising outcomes, reflecting advancements in biomaterial technology and surgical techniques. Our study presents compelling evidence supporting the capabilities of PLGA implants in maintaining functional ROM while minimizing complications, thereby enhancing the overall recovery experience for young patients.

5. Conclusions

Our study demonstrates that PLGA intramedullary implants effectively restore function and ensure proper bone healing in pediatric diaphyseal forearm fractures. Children showed only a minor reduction in mobility, indicating the precision of these implants in preserving a near-normal ROM. Consistent functional outcomes across different ages, genders, and fracture types highlight the versatility of PLGA implants. They offer a patient-friendly alternative to traditional metallic implants, which often require removal surgeries and pose long-term risks such as hardware irritation or migration. The biodegradable nature of PLGA eliminates the need for a second surgery, reducing healthcare burdens and psychological impacts on young patients and their families while decreasing anesthesia-related risks and peri- and postoperative complications such as vessel or nerve injuries, infections, or scar tissue formation. Additionally, fewer hospital stays and follow-up visits minimize disruptions to a child's education and social life, crucial for their development. While PLGA's degradation process may introduce some intermediary byproducts, the overall benefits seem to outweigh these concerns.

Future research should focus on the long-term effects of PLGA implants on bone health and growth, expanding to larger, diverse populations to validate findings. Additionally, investigating the economic impact and exploring their application in other pediatric orthopedic conditions could further substantiate PLGA implants' adoption in clinical practice. Currently, PLGA implants represent a significant advancement in pediatric fracture management, enhancing recovery experiences for young patients.

Author Contributions: Conceptualization, A.L., Á.M.L. and G.J.; methodology, A.K., A.L., G.J. and H.N.; software, A.K., A.L. and H.N.; validation, A.K., A.L., Á.M.L., H.N. and G.J.; formal analysis, A.K., A.L., Á.M.L. and H.N.; investigation, Á.M.L., H.N. and G.J.; resources, G.J.; data curation, A.K., A.L., Á.M.L. and H.N.; writing—original draft preparation, A.L.; writing—review and editing, A.K., Á.M.L., A.L., G.J. and H.N.; visualization, A.K., A.L. and H.N.; supervision, A.K., A.L. and G.J.; project administration, A.K., A.L. and G.J.; funding acquisition, G.J. All authors have read and agreed to the published version of the manuscript.

Funding: This research received no external funding. All resources were funded by the University of Pécs, Medical School.

Institutional Review Board Statement: The study was conducted according to the guidelines of the Declaration of Helsinki and approved by the Regional Research Ethics Committee, Clinical Complex, University of Pécs (Pécsi Tudományegyetem, Klinikai Komplex, Regionális és Intézményi Kutatás—Etikai Bizottság) on 23 April 2021 (8737-PTE2021).

Informed Consent Statement: Informed consent was obtained from all subjects involved in the study. Written informed consent was obtained from the guardians of the patients to publish this paper.

Data Availability Statement: All data are contained within the article.

Conflicts of Interest: The authors declare no conflicts of interest.

References

1. Naranje, S.M.; Erali, R.A.; Warner, W.C.J.; Sawyer, J.R.; Kelly, D.M. Epidemiology of Pediatric Fractures Presenting to Emergency Departments in the United States. *J. Pediatr. Orthop.* **2016**, *36*, e45. [CrossRef]
2. Chia, B.; Kozin, S.H.; Herman, M.J.; Safier, S.; Abzug, J.M. Complications of Pediatric Distal Radius and Forearm Fractures. *Instr. Course Lect.* **2015**, *64*, 499–507. [PubMed]
3. Salvi, A.E. Forearm Diaphyseal Fractures: Which Bone to Synthesize First? *Orthopedics* **2006**, *29*, 669–671, discussion 671. [CrossRef] [PubMed]
4. Manson, T.T.; Pfaeffle, H.J.; Herdon, J.H.; Tomaino, M.M.; Fischer, K.J. Forearm Rotation Alters Interosseous Ligament Strain Distribution. *J. Hand Surg.* **2000**, *25*, 1058–1063. [CrossRef] [PubMed]
5. Widnall, J.; Bruce, C. Paediatric Forearm Fractures. *Orthop. Trauma* **2018**, *32*, 372–377. [CrossRef]
6. Noonan, K.J.; Price, C.T. Forearm and Distal Radius Fractures in Children. *J. Am. Acad. Orthop. Surg.* **1998**, *6*, 146–156. [CrossRef] [PubMed]
7. Epema, A.C.; Spanjer, M.J.B.; Ras, L.; Kelder, J.C.; Sanders, M. Point-of-Care Ultrasound Compared with Conventional Radiographic Evaluation in Children with Suspected Distal Forearm Fractures in the Netherlands: A Diagnostic Accuracy Study. *Emerg. Med. J. EMJ* **2019**, *36*, 613–616. [CrossRef]
8. Caruso, G.; Caldari, E.; Sturla, F.D.; Caldaria, A.; Re, D.L.; Pagetti, P.; Palummieri, F.; Massari, L. Management of Pediatric Forearm Fractures: What Is the Best Therapeutic Choice? A Narrative Review of the Literature. *Musculoskelet. Surg.* **2021**, *105*, 225–234. [CrossRef] [PubMed]
9. The AO Pediatric Comprehensive Classification of Long Bone Fractures (PCCF) | Acta Orthopaedica. Available online: https://actaorthop.org/actao/article/view/9669 (accessed on 31 May 2024).
10. Randsborg, P.-H.; Sivertsen, E.A. Distal Radius Fractures in Children: Substantial Difference in Stability between Buckle and Greenstick Fractures. *Acta Orthop.* **2009**, *80*, 585–589. [CrossRef]
11. Atanelov, Z.; Bentley, T.P. Greenstick Fracture. In *StatPearls*; StatPearls Publishing: Treasure Island, FL, USA, 2024.
12. Poutoglidou, F. Flexible Intramedullary Nailing in the Treatment of Forearm Fractures in Children and Adolescents, a Systematic Review. *J. Orthop.* **2020**, *20*, 125–130. [CrossRef]
13. Flynn, J.M.; Jones, K.J.; Garner, M.R.; Goebel, J. Eleven Years Experience in the Operative Management of Pediatric Forearm Fractures. *J. Pediatr. Orthop.* **2010**, *30*, 313–319. [CrossRef] [PubMed]
14. Lascombes, P.; Prevot, J.; Ligier, J.N.; Metaizeau, J.P.; Poncelet, T. Elastic Stable Intramedullary Nailing in Forearm Shaft Fractures in Children: 85 Cases. *J. Pediatr. Orthop.* **1990**, *10*, 167–171. [CrossRef] [PubMed]
15. Heye, P.; Matissek, C.; Seidl, C.; Varga, M.; Kassai, T.; Jozsa, G.; Krebs, T. Making Hardware Removal Unnecessary by Using Resorbable Implants for Osteosynthesis in Children. *Children* **2022**, *9*, 471. [CrossRef] [PubMed]
16. Roeder, C.; Alves, C.; Balslev-Clausen, A.; Canavese, F.; Gercek, E.; Kassai, T.; Klestil, T.; Klingenberg, L.; Lutz, N.; Varga, M.; et al. Pilot Study and Preliminary Results of Biodegradable Intramedullary Nailing of Forearm Fractures in Children. *Children* **2022**, *9*, 754. [CrossRef] [PubMed]

17. Perhomaa, M.; Pokka, T.; Korhonen, L.; Kyrö, A.; Niinimäki, J.; Serlo, W.; Sinikumpu, J.-J. Randomized Controlled Trial of the Clinical Recovery and Biodegradation of Polylactide-Co-Glycolide Implants Used in the Intramedullary Nailing of Children's Forearm Shaft Fractures with at Least Four Years of Follow-Up. *J. Clin. Med.* **2021**, *10*, 995. [CrossRef]
18. Helber, M.U.; Ulrich, C. External Fixation in Forearm Shaft Fractures. *Injury* **2000**, *31* (Suppl. S1), 45–47. [CrossRef] [PubMed]
19. Elhalawany, A.S.; Afifi, A.; Anbar, A.; Galal, S. Hybrid Fixation for Adolescent Both-Bones Diaphyseal Forearm Fractures: Preliminary Results of a Prospective Cohort Study. *J. Clin. Orthop. Trauma* **2020**, *11*, S46–S50. [CrossRef] [PubMed]
20. Korhonen, L.; Perhomaa, M.; Kyrö, A.; Pokka, T.; Serlo, W.; Merikanto, J.; Sinikumpu, J.-J. Intramedullary Nailing of Forearm Shaft Fractures by Biodegradable Compared with Titanium Nails: Results of a Prospective Randomized Trial in Children with at Least Two Years of Follow-Up. *Biomaterials* **2018**, *185*, 383–392. [CrossRef]
21. Varga, M.; Józsa, G.; Hanna, D.; Tóth, M.; Hajnal, B.; Krupa, Z.; Kassai, T. Bioresorbable Implants vs. Kirschner-Wires in the Treatment of Severely Displaced Distal Paediatric Radius and Forearm Fractures—A Retrospective Multicentre Study. *BMC Musculoskelet. Disord.* **2022**, *23*, 362. [CrossRef]
22. von Elm, E.; Altman, D.G.; Egger, M.; Pocock, S.J.; Gøtzsche, P.C.; Vandenbroucke, J.P. The Strengthening the Reporting of Observational Studies in Epidemiology (STROBE) Statement: Guidelines for Reporting Observational Studies. *J. Clin. Epidemiol.* **2008**, *61*, 344–349. [CrossRef]
23. Gentile, P.; Chiono, V.; Carmagnola, I.; Hatton, P.V. An Overview of Poly(Lactic-Co-Glycolic) Acid (PLGA)-Based Biomaterials for Bone Tissue Engineering. *Int. J. Mol. Sci.* **2014**, *15*, 3640–3659. [CrossRef] [PubMed]
24. Engineer, C.; Parikh, J.; Raval, A. Review on Hydrolytic Degradation Behavior of Biodegradable Polymers from Controlled Drug Delivery System. *Trends Biomater. Artif. Organs* **2011**, *25*, 79–85.
25. Eppley, B.L.; Reilly, M. Degradation Characteristics of PLLA-PGA Bone Fixation Devices. *J. Craniofac. Surg.* **1997**, *8*, 116. [CrossRef] [PubMed]
26. Fearmonti, R.; Bond, J.; Erdmann, D.; Levinson, H. A Review of Scar Scales and Scar Measuring Devices. *Eplasty* **2010**, *10*, e43. [PubMed]
27. Chereddy, K.K.; Payen, V.L.; Préat, V. PLGA: From a Classic Drug Carrier to a Novel Therapeutic Activity Contributor. *J. Control. Release* **2018**, *289*, 10–13. [CrossRef] [PubMed]
28. Żywicka, B.; Krucińska, I.; Garcarek, J.; Szymonowicz, M.; Komisarczyk, A.; Rybak, Z. Biological Properties of Low-Toxic PLGA and PLGA/PHB Fibrous Nanocomposite Scaffolds for Osseous Tissue Regeneration. Evaluation of Potential Bioactivity. *Molecules* **2017**, *22*, 1852. [CrossRef]
29. Paterson, N.; Waterhouse, P. Risk in Pediatric Anesthesia: Risk in Pediatric Anesthesia. *Pediatr. Anesth.* **2011**, *21*, 848–857. [CrossRef] [PubMed]
30. Józsa, G.; Kassai, T.; Varga, M. Preliminary Experience with Bioabsorbable Intramedullary Nails for Paediatric Forearm Fractures: Results of a Mini-Series. *Genij Ortop.* **2023**, *29*, 640–644. [CrossRef]
31. Nudelman, H.; Lőrincz, A.; Lamberti, A.G.; Varga, M.; Kassai, T.; Józsa, G. Management of Juvenile Osteochondral Fractures Utilising Absorbable PLGA Implants. *J. Clin. Med.* **2024**, *13*, 375. [CrossRef]
32. Válik, A.; Harangozó, K.; Garami, A.; Juhász, Z.; Józsa, G.; Lőrincz, A. Mid-Term Follow-Up Study of Children Undergoing Autologous Skin Transplantation for Burns. *Life* **2023**, *13*, 762. [CrossRef]
33. Navratilova, P.; Emmer, J.; Tomas, T.; Ryba, L.; Burda, J.; Loja, T.; Veverkova, J.; Valkova, L.; Pavkova Goldbergova, M. Plastic Response of Macrophages to Metal Ions and Nanoparticles in Time Mimicking Metal Implant Body Environment. *Environ. Sci. Pollut. Res.* **2024**, *31*, 4111–4129. [CrossRef]
34. Sun, C.W.Y.; Lau, L.C.M.; Cheung, J.P.Y.; Choi, S.-W. Cancer-Causing Effects of Orthopaedic Metal Implants in Total Hip Arthroplasty. *Cancers* **2024**, *16*, 1339. [CrossRef] [PubMed]
35. Hedelin, H.; Larnert, P.; Antonsson, P.; Lagerstrand, K.; Brisby, H.; Hebelka, H.; Laine, T. Stability in Pelvic Triple Osteotomies in Children Using Resorbable PLGA Screws for Fixation. *J. Pediatr. Orthop.* **2021**, *41*, e787–e792. [CrossRef]
36. Landes, C.A.; Ballon, A.; Roth, C. Maxillary and Mandibular Osteosyntheses with PLGA and P(L/DL)LA Implants: A 5-Year Inpatient Biocompatibility and Degradation Experience. *Plast. Reconstr. Surg.* **2006**, *117*, 2347–2360. [CrossRef]
37. Xu, L.; Fukumura, D.; Jain, R.K. Acidic Extracellular pH Induces Vascular Endothelial Growth Factor (VEGF) in Human Glioblastoma Cells via ERK1/2 MAPK Signaling Pathway: Mechanism of low pH-induced VEGF. *J. Biol. Chem.* **2002**, *277*, 11368–11374. [CrossRef] [PubMed]
38. Davis, R.; Singh, A.; Jackson, M.J.; Coelho, R.T.; Prakash, D.; Charalambous, C.P.; Ahmed, W.; da Silva, L.R.R.; Lawrence, A.A. A Comprehensive Review on Metallic Implant Biomaterials and Their Subtractive Manufacturing. *Int. J. Adv. Manuf. Technol.* **2022**, *120*, 1473–1530. [CrossRef] [PubMed]
39. Wall, L.; O'Donnell, J.C.; Schoenecker, P.L.; Keeler, K.A.; Dobbs, M.B.; Luhmann, S.J.; Gordon, J.E. Titanium Elastic Nailing Radius and Ulna Fractures in Adolescents. *J. Pediatr. Orthop. Part B* **2012**, *21*, 482–488. [CrossRef]
40. Patel, A.; Li, L.; Anand, A. Systematic Review: Functional Outcomes and Complications of Intramedullary Nailing versus Plate Fixation for Both-Bone Diaphyseal Forearm Fractures in Children. *Injury* **2014**, *45*, 1135–1143. [CrossRef]

41. Martus, J.E.; Preston, R.K.; Schoenecker, J.G.; Lovejoy, S.A.; Green, N.E.; Mencio, G.A. Complications and Outcomes of Diaphyseal Forearm Fracture Intramedullary Nailing: A Comparison of Pediatric and Adolescent Age Groups. *J. Pediatr. Orthop.* **2013**, *33*, 598. [CrossRef]
42. Jaspers, M.E.H.; Moortgat, P. Objective Assessment Tools: Physical Parameters in Scar Assessment. In *Textbook on Scar Management: State of the Art Management and Emerging Technologies*; Téot, L., Mustoe, T.A., Middelkoop, E., Gauglitz, G.G., Eds.; Springer: Cham, Switzerland, 2020; ISBN 978-3-030-44765-6.

Journal of
Clinical Medicine

MDPI

Article

Stress Analysis in Conversion Total Hip Arthroplasty: A Finite Element Analysis on Stem Length and Distal Screw Hole

Koshiro Shimasaki, Tomofumi Nishino *, Tomohiro Yoshizawa, Ryunosuke Watanabe, Fumi Hirose, Shota Yasunaga and Hajime Mishima

Department of Orthopaedic Surgery, Institute of Medicine, University of Tsukuba, 1-1-1, Tennodai, Tsukuba 305-8575, Ibaraki, Japan; koshiro19881020@tsukuba-seikei.jp (K.S.); tyoshizawa@tsukuba-seikei.jp (T.Y.); ryuwatanabe@tsukuba-seikei.jp (R.W.); f.ochiai.0023@tsukuba-seikei.jp (F.H.); syasunaga@tsukuba-seikei.jp (S.Y.); hmishima@tsukuba-seikei.jp (H.M.)

* Correspondence: nishino@tsukuba-seikei.jp; Tel.: +81-029-853-7668; Fax: +81-029-853-3712

Abstract: Background/Objectives: Proximal femoral fractures are particularly common in older adults, and cases requiring conversion to total hip arthroplasty may arise because of treatment failure or osteoarthritis. Fractures around the distal screw removal holes can be problematic. This study aimed to analyze the relationship between stem length and femoral stress distribution to determine the optimal stem length. **Methods:** A finite element analysis simulation was conducted using pre-existing femoral computed tomography data, an intramedullary nail, and three types of stems of varying lengths. Loads simulating normal walking and stair climbing were applied, and the average and maximum equivalent stresses were measured on both the medial and lateral sides of the distal screw removal hole for each stem length. Statistical analysis was then performed to evaluate the stress distributions. **Results:** The average stress around the distal screw removal hole tended to decrease as stem length increased. The maximum stress was significantly lower with the 160-mm stem, which provides a 40-mm bridging length, compared to the 120-mm and 130-mm stems, where the stem tip aligned with or only slightly extended past the distal screw removal hole (bridging lengths of 0 mm and 10 mm, respectively). **Conclusions:** In conversion hip total arthroplasty following proximal femoral fractures, using a sufficiently long stem can help avoid stress concentration around the distal screw removal hole, thereby potentially reducing the risk of periprosthetic fractures.

Keywords: osteoporosis; femoral trochanteric fracture; conversion total hip arthroplasty; periprosthetic fracture; stress distribution

1. Introduction

Proximal femoral fractures, which are particularly common in older adults, are frequently managed surgically using intramedullary nails, especially in those with unstable fracture patterns, as indicated by the American and British guidelines [1,2]. However, complications such as cut-out, nonunion, and pseudarthrosis, or conditions like femoral head necrosis and osteoarthritis, may necessitate salvage surgery, specifically conversion to total hip arthroplasty (cTHA) [3–6]. Compared to primary THA, cTHA is more complex, complicated by proximal femur nonunion, bone defects, poor bone quality, reduced offset, bone sclerosis around prior hardware removal sites, and challenges in fracture fixation and stem selection [7–11].

Consequently, cTHA involves longer surgery times, greater blood loss [7,12–15], and a higher risk of complications, including dislocation (11.4%), periprosthetic fractures (6.2%),

https://doi.org/10.3390/jcm14010106

and infection (3.8%) [8,15,16]. The 1-year mortality rate post-cTHA has also been reported at 13.6% [13,14,17–20]. With the growing older adult population and increased incidence of femoral fractures, the demand for cTHA and attention to its associated risks are expected to increase.

Periprosthetic fractures during cTHA are classified as intraoperative or postoperative. Intraoperatively, fractures often occur around the proximal femur, such as in the greater trochanter or calcar region [7–11], owing to surgical stress from reaming or stem insertion, particularly in osteoporotic or previously deformed bones, leading to iatrogenic fractures [8,21]. Postoperatively, fractures are observed not only in the proximal femur but also around the distal screw removal holes [14,22–24], often resulting from long-term osteolysis or stem loosening [25], or in the short term from stress concentration at the distal stem [26,27], often occurring without significant trauma [28,29].

Cortical holes left by previous screws should ideally be plugged during surgery whenever possible. This is because these holes can lead to inadequate cement pressurization when using a cemented stem and serve as potential sites for stress concentration, increasing the risk of femoral fracture when using a cementless stem [8].

In terms of stem length, short stems have the advantage of preserving bone stock and achieving a more physiological distribution of femoral stress. However, in patients with poor bone quality and limited bone stock, there is concern about the risk of periprosthetic fractures around the stem due to increased stress on the bone. On the other hand, long stems are expected to reduce the risk of localized stress concentration through higher stress distribution effects and greater stiffness than short stems. Nevertheless, stress shielding in the proximal region can be a significant issue, and if the load is not transmitted through the proximal femur, proximal bone loss is inevitable [30–32].

While some reports argue that extensive bridging over screw removal holes is unnecessary [33], many surgeons favor the use of long revision stems [8,11,34–38], particularly with cortical defects, and recommend a bridging length of approximately two femoral diameters (approximately 40 mm) [39–41]. However, the optimal bridging length and the effects of stem length on the stress distribution around screw removal holes remain under-researched, with no consensus on best practices.

Currently, there are reports indicating that there is no difference in clinical outcomes for cTHA depending on the stem used or techniques employed for bone fixation. Therefore, from the perspective of femoral stress distribution, it is considered practical to use either a cementless long stem or a cemented stem in clinical practice. From the perspective of risks, such as insufficient cement injection pressure due to multiple implant removal holes and the risk of BCIS (Bone Cement Implantation syndrome), the use of cementless stems is appealing.

We, therefore, aimed to analyze the stress distribution around the distal screw removal hole during cTHA following proximal femoral fractures and determine the optimal stem length. Simulations were conducted using finite element analysis (FEA) with stems of varying lengths. Our hypothesis was that the stress concentration would peak when the stem tip was aligned with the distal screw removal hole. Furthermore, considering that a bridging length of at least twice the femoral diameter is recommended for fractures or large cortical defects [39–41], we hypothesized that a length of 1.5 × the femoral diameter may significantly reduce stress around the screw removal hole.

2. Materials and Methods

Informed consent was obtained from the patient for the use and publication of the data. This analytical observational study was approved by the Ethics Review Committee of our institution (approval code: H27-041). This analytical observational study utilized existing computed tomography (CT) and femoral implant Standard Triangulated Language (STL) data to conduct FEA simulations. We then aimed to analyze the stress distribution in the femur.

Before starting this study, we calculated the required sample size using the statistical power analysis software, G*Power (version 3.1.9.7; University of Düsseldorf, Düsseldorf, Germany). Assuming an effect size of 0.25, a significance level of 0.05, a power of 0.8, and three groups for the parametric test, the minimum required sample size was determined to be 28. Based on this, we decided to analyze 30 cases (30 limbs) of femoral CT data. The population from which the sample data were drawn consisted of 100 female patients aged 75 or younger who underwent their first total hip arthroplasty at our institution between October 2021 and September 2024, all classified as Dorr Type B [42]. Patients with a history of femoral osteotomy or severe deformities, such as Perthes-like deformities, were excluded. Thirty patients (30 limbs) were randomly selected for analysis to minimize selection bias and improve statistical power, thereby enhancing the reliability and validity of the study results.

Femoral CT data were obtained from the unaffected side. Because CT imaging conditions were standardized during the study period, data quality was sufficiently ensured, and selection bias related to the period was negligible. One of the evaluation methods for femoral morphology, the Dorr classification, involves a subjective assessment. In this study, three experienced orthopedic surgeons independently evaluated the preoperative plain radiographs and classified the femoral morphology as Type A, B, or C. The intraclass correlation coefficient (ICC) was used to assess inter-rater reliability, yielding an ICC of 0.80 (95% CI: 0.72–0.88), demonstrating high consistency among the raters. Therefore, we confirmed that the Dorr classification used in this study has sufficient reliability.

CT data used in this study were obtained using a 256-slice multidetector CT scanner (Brilliance iCT; Philips Healthcare, Cleveland, OH, USA). The femur was scanned from the pelvis to both knee joints, along with a bone density phantom (QRM-BDC/3 Phantom, QRM Quality Assurance in Radiology and Medicine GmbH, Möhrendorf, Germany) under conditions of 120 kV/166 mAs and 1 mm slice thickness.

The FEA analysis software used was MECHANICAL FINDER (MF, version 13.0, Extended Edition, Research Center of Computational Mechanics, Tokyo, Japan), which constructs a heterogeneous material model based on bone density derived from CT values and allows for detailed stress and strength analysis. First, the CT data were imported into the MF, and a three-dimensional (3D) femoral model of the unaffected side was constructed. Next, a femoral model was created after screw removal (removal model). In this study, a 3D–3D registration was performed on the healthy femur model and the STL data of the intramedullary nail in MF, and the material properties of the nail were set to "unused" to replace the nail with a void, thus recreating the femur after screw removal.

The intramedullary nail used was the Trochanteric Fixation Nail Advanced (TFNA) Proximal Femoral Nailing System (Depuy Synthes, Raynham, MA, USA), represented by φ10 mm × 200 mm/130° STL data. The distal screw was 5 mm long and designed to be 135 mm from the proximal end of the nail. The screw was inserted into the 3D femoral model such that the tip-apex distance was <20 mm, with the distal screw fixed statically at a diameter of 5 mm. The stem used was a Universia stem (Teijin Nakashima Medical, Okayama, Japan) #11, high offset, in the STL format. The Universia stem is designed to fit the femoral morphology of the Japanese population and is a cementless stem coated with hydroxyapatite on all surfaces [43].

The STL data from the Universia stem were inserted into the removal model to create a cTHA model (Figure 1). The stems were divided based on their length into three groups: (1) short (120 mm stem, hereafter referred to as the S group); (2) normal (130 mm stem,

N group); and (3) long (160 mm stem, L group) (Figure 1). In clinical practice, the 130 mm normal stem is the only one used, whereas the short and long stems were newly constructed virtual stems for this simulation. The long stem was selected based on previous studies that recommended a bridging length of approximately 40 mm for fractures or large cortical bone defects [39–41], and a stem length of 160 mm was used for verification.

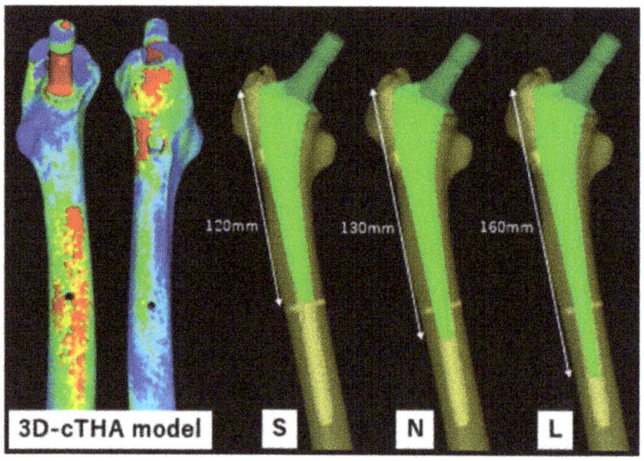

Figure 1. 3D-cTHA model, constructed by inserting a stem into a 3D femoral model after intramedullary nail removal. Three types of stems were used: a short stem (S, 120 mm) with its tip at the same level as the distal screw extraction hole; a normal stem (N, 130 mm) bridging 10 mm beyond the hole; and a long stem (L, 160 mm) bridging 40 mm.

Simulations were conducted under a load to analyze the femoral stress distribution for each stem length. The femoral neck osteotomy and stem placement positions were initially planned using the 3D preoperative planning software, ZedHip (version 17.0.0; Lexi Co., Ltd., Tokyo, Japan) (Figure 2) and were faithfully reproduced in the MF.

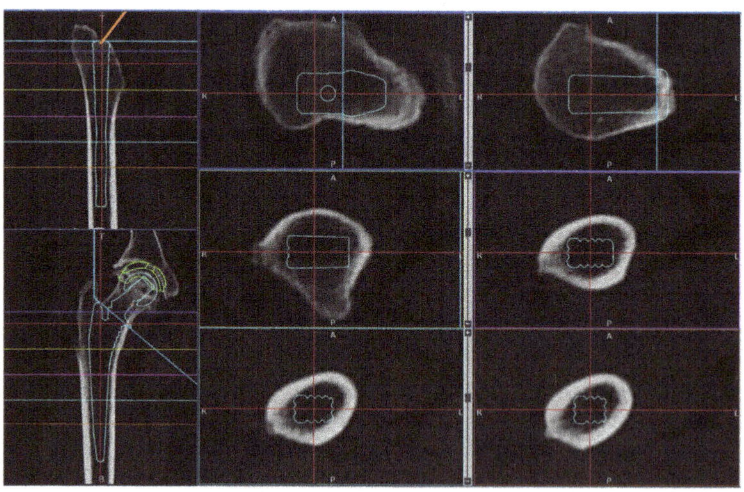

Figure 2. Preparation for cTHA. Preoperative planning was performed using the 3D preoperative planning software, ZedHip (version 17.0.0; Lexi Co., Ltd., Tokyo, Japan).

2.1. Material Parameters

Solid elements with 4-node tetrahedral elements were used in this study. A shell element with a thickness of 0.001 mm, which did not influence the strength, was applied to the bone surface. A mesh convergence test was conducted to determine the mesh size (Figure 3).

To determine an appropriate mesh size for the finite element analysis, a mesh convergence test was conducted. Several mesh sizes were evaluated, and the resulting stress values were compared to identify the point at which further refinement caused a change of less than 1%. Based on these results, an optimal mesh size was selected to balance computational efficiency and solution accuracy. This approach ensured that the analysis provided reliable results while minimizing unnecessary computational costs.

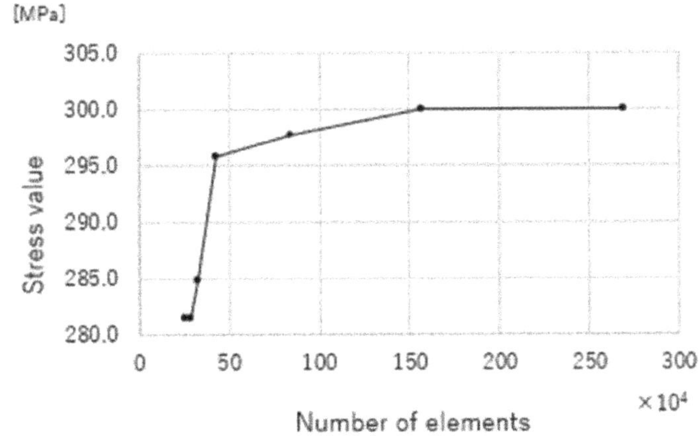

Figure 3. Mesh convergence test. The optimal mesh size was determined by confirming the conditions under which the stress variation remained below 1%. This choice balances the analysis precision and computational efficiency, allowing high accuracy while minimizing the calculation time.

An inhomogeneous material model was used for the bones. Young's modulus was calculated from the bone mineral density (BMD, ρ [g/cm^3]) based on the CT values (Hounsfield Units: HU) using a linear relationship [44,45]. Subsequently, the values were estimated using Keyak's predictive transformation formula and incorporated into the model [46]. Poisson's ratio was set as 0.40 [44,46]. The stem was modeled using a homogeneous material model with the material properties of a titanium alloy (Ti-6Al-4V), Young's modulus of 109 GPa, and Poisson's ratio of 0.28 [44,46] (Table 1).

Table 1. Material parameters.

	Materials	Young's Modulus [GPa]	Poisson's Ratio
Femoral bone	Heterogeneous model	Keyak (1998) [46]	0.40
Stem	Titanium alloy (Ti-6Al-4V)	109	0.28

2.2. Loading and Boundary Conditions

The loading conditions were based on the maximum load during daily activities. For this study, maximum loads during "normal walking" and "stair climbing" were adopted, based on previous reports [47,48]. The loads are shown in Table 2 and Figure 4, and the magnitude of each vector was determined based on the weight of the patient. The boundary conditions were set for full restraint at the distal femur (Figure 4), and the contact condition between the femur and stem was defined with a friction coefficient of 0.49 [49].

Table 2. Loading conditions.

Force	X (N)	Y (N)	Z (N)	Acting Point	%
Normal Walking					
Hip contact	Lt. 54.0/Rt. −54.0	32.8	−229.2	P0	238
ABD	Lt. 58.0/Rt. −58.0	4.3	86.5	P1	104
TFL-P	Lt. 7.2/Rt. −7.2	11.6	13.2	P1	19
TFL-D	Lt. −0.5/Rt. 0.5	−0.7	−19.0	P1	19
P1 total force	Lt. −64.7/Rt. 64.7	−15.2	80.7	P1	105
VL	Lt. −0.9/Rt. 0.9	−18.5	−92.9	P2	95
Stair climbing					
Force	**X (N)**	**Y (N)**	**Z (N)**	**Acting point**	**%**
Hip contact	Lt. 59.3/Rt. −59.3	60.6	−236.3	P0	251
ABD	Lt. 70.1/Rt. −70.1	28.8	84.9	P1	
ITT-P	Lt. 10.5/Rt. −10.5	3.0	12.8	P1	
ITT-D	Lt. −0.5/Rt. 0.5	−0.8	−16.8	P1	
TFL-P	Lt. 3.1/Rt. −3.1	4.9	2.9	P1	
TFL-D	Lt. −0.2/Rt. 0.2	−0.3	−6.5	P1	
P1 total force	Lt. −83.0/Rt. 83.0	−35.6	77.3	P1	119
VL	Lt. −2.2/Rt. 2.2	−22.4	−135.1	P2	137
VM	Lt. −8.8/Rt. 8.8	−39.6	−267.1	P3	270

ABD, Abductor; TFL, Tensor Fascia Latae; TFL-P, Tensor Fascia Latae-Proximal; TFL-D, Tensor Fascia Latae-Distal; VL, Vastus Lateralis; VM, Vastus Medialis.

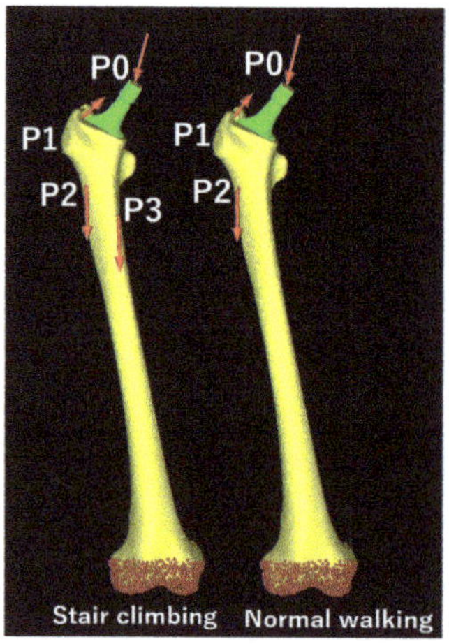

Figure 4. Loading conditions. Loading points and fixation sites for simulated normal climbing and stair climbing. P0, hip contact point; P1, a combined force of the abductor muscles and iliotibial band; P2, action point of the vastus lateralis; P3, action point of the vastus medialis. The distal femur was fully constrained under both conditions.

2.3. Static Structural Analysis

The load was applied linearly, and an elastic analysis was performed. The calculations were performed using linear static analysis.

2.4. Data Collection and Candidate Predictors

Patient background data included age (years), height (m), weight (kg), BMI (kg/m^2), femoral neck BMD (g/cm^2), and Canal Flare Index (CFI) [50]. Preoperative measurements of age, height, weight, BMI, and BMD were assessed using a Hologic Discovery A scanner

(Hologic Inc., Bedford, MA, USA). Additionally, the parameters of the constructed cTHA model, such as the stem anteversion angle (°), bridging length (mm), and distal screw length (mm), were measured. To ensure intra-observer reliability, each parameter was measured three times under the same conditions, and the average of these measurements was used for the final data. All data were expressed as mean ± standard deviation (SD).

2.5. Outcomes

Simulations were performed for the S, N, and L groups during "normal walking" and "stair climbing", and a linear analysis was used to calculate the average and maximum stress values on the medial and lateral sides of the distal screw removal hole. The study area was defined as the bone surface shell elements within a 10-mm radius sphere centered around the distal screw removal hole (Figure 5). The equivalent stress [MPa] was used, and all data were expressed as mean (95% CI).

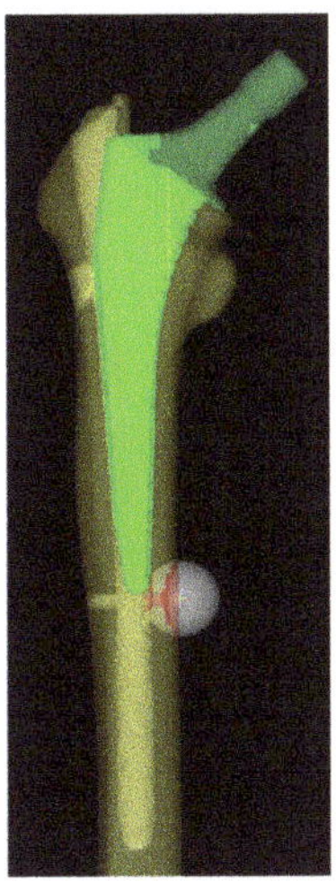

Figure 5. Regions of interest for stress value calculations. The target area of investigation was defined as the shell elements of the bone surface within a spherical region with a 10-mm radius centered on the distal screw removal hole.

2.6. Statistical Analysis

Statistical analysis of the maximum equivalent stress around the distal screw removal hole was performed using SPSS Statistics version 29 (IBM Corp., Armonk, NY, USA). The normality of the data was assessed using the Shapiro–Wilk test. A significance level of $\alpha = 0.05$ was set; if the p-value exceeded 0.05, the data were considered normally distributed, and an appropriate statistical test to compare the three groups was selected.

3. Results

3.1. Flow Chart of Patients

Patient flow in this study is shown in Figure 6.

First, out of a total of 231 patients who underwent THA at our institution between October 2021 and September 2024, we identified 132 cases involving women aged 75 or younger with Dorr classification type B. Among these, 11 cases with a history of femoral surgery and 21 cases with severe deformities such as Perthes-like deformities were excluded, leaving 100 eligible cases. From these 100 cases, 30 were selected using a simple random sampling method, and the contralateral femoral CT data from these patients were used for analysis.

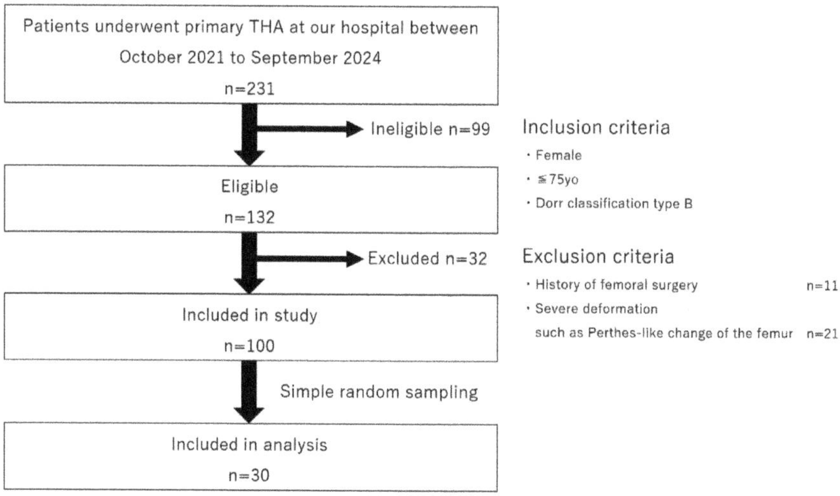

Figure 6. Flowchart of study data selection, including patient recruitment and exclusion criteria.

3.2. Characteristics of Patients and 3D-cTHA Model

The characteristics of the patients and the 3D-cTHA model used in this study are summarized in Table 3.

Table 3. Patient characteristics and 3D-cTHA model.

Characteristic	Value
Age (mean ± SD) [years]	66.5 ± 8.7
Hight (mean ± SD) [m]	1.53 ± 0.06
Body weight (mean ± SD) [kg]	53.5 ± 9.0
Body mass index (mean ± SD) [kg/m^2]	22.7 ± 3.2
Side [limb]	Left 16; Right 14
Bone mineral density of the femoral neck (mean ± SD) [g/cm^2]	0.61 ± 0.13
Canal flare index (mean ± SD)	4.17 ± 0.42
Length of distal screw (mean ± SD) [mm]	25.7 ± 1.7
Femoral anteversion (mean ± SD) [degrees]	21.69 ± 10.69

3.3. Analysis

The maximum equivalent stress values at the medial and lateral sides of the distal screw removal hole during "normal walking" and "stair climbing" for the three groups (S, N, and L) were confirmed to follow a normal distribution. The normality tests for each group showed: "normal walking" (medial side: S group, W = 0.949, p = 0.155; N group, W = 0.947, p = 0.140; L group, W = 0.980, p = 0.830; lateral side: S group, W = 0.976, p = 0.702; N group, W = 0.975, p = 0.690; L group, W = 0.967, p = 0.465); "stair climbing" (medial side: S group, W = 0.963, p = 0.378; N group, W = 0.973, p = 0.612; L group, W = 0.970; p = 0.548; lateral side: S group, W = 0.965, p = 0.403; N group, W = 0.957, p = 0.259; L group, W = 0.981, p = 0.844) (Figure 7).

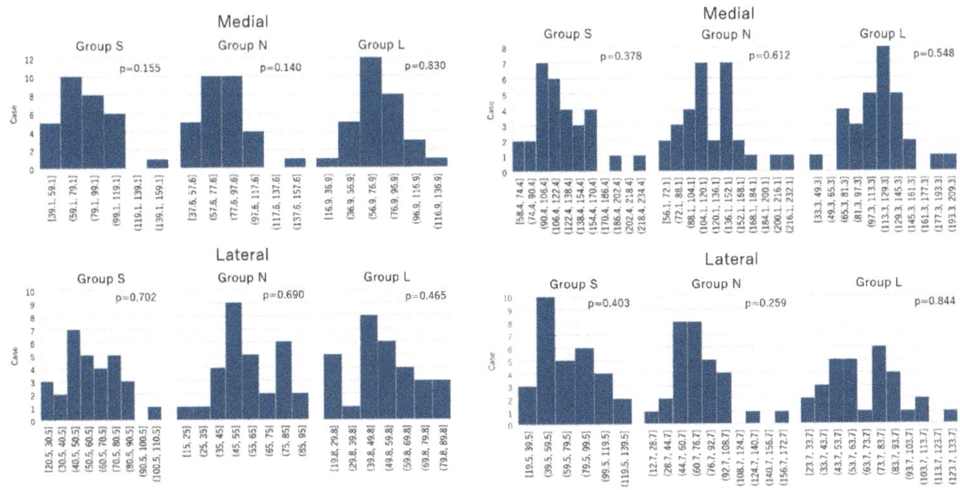

(a) (b)

Figure 7. Histogram of the normality test performed using the Shapiro–Wilk test. (**a**) Normal walking; (**b**) Stair climbing. The collected data followed a normal distribution under both the normal and stair-climbing conditions.

Based on these results, repeated measures analysis of variance (ANOVA) was used to compare the three groups. The Bonferroni correction was applied for post-hoc multiple comparisons, and pairwise differences between all three groups were evaluated.

3.4. Mean Equivalent Stress Around the Distal Screw Removal Hole

A scatter plot of the mean equivalent stress values at the distal screw removal hole for different stem lengths and fitted lines is shown in Figure 8. Both during "normal walking" and "stair climbing", the mean equivalent stress decreased with increasing stem length.

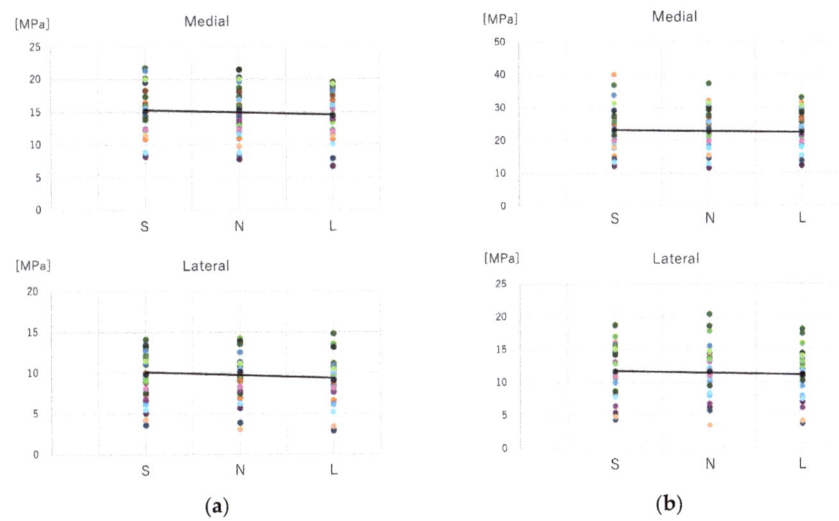

(a) (b)

Figure 8. Comparison of average values of equivalent stress. (**a**) Normal walking; (**b**) Stair climbing. Under both normal walking and stair climbing conditions, the average stress around the distal screw removal hole tended to decrease as the stem length increased.

3.5. Maximum Equivalent Stress Around the Distal Screw Removal Hole

3.5.1. Normal Walking

a. Comparison between groups

For the medial side, the stress was 79.9 (95% CI: 70.8–89.0) MPa for the S group, 79.6 (95% CI: 70.5–88.8) MPa for the N group, and 73.2 (95% CI: 64.9–81.6) MPa for the L group. For the lateral side, it was 58.4 (95% CI: 50.9–65.9) MPa for the S group, 58.5 (95% CI: 51.5–65.5) MPa for the N group, and 52.9 (95% CI: 46.0–59.8) MPa for the L group. Both medial and lateral sides showed significant main effects in the analysis of variance (medial side: F (2, 58) = 9.940, $p < 0.001$, $\eta^2 = 0.26$; lateral side: F (2, 58) = 8.311, $p < 0.001$, $\eta^2 = 0.22$) (Figure 9).

b. Post-hoc multiple comparisons

Significant differences were found between the S and L groups and the N and L groups on both the medial and lateral sides (S vs. L: medial, $p = 0.006$; lateral, $p = 0.004$; N vs. L, medial $p = 0.003$, lateral $p = 0.005$). On the medial side, the stress in the S group was 6.67 MPa higher than that in the L group (95% CI: 1.69–11.64), and 6.40 MPa higher than that in the N group (95% CI: 1.96–10.83). On the lateral side, the S group showed 5.52 MPa higher stress than the L group (95% CI: 1.53–9.50) and 5.50 MPa higher than the N group (95% CI: 1.48–9.52). No significant differences were found between the S and N groups (medial and lateral: $p > 0.99$) (Figure 9).

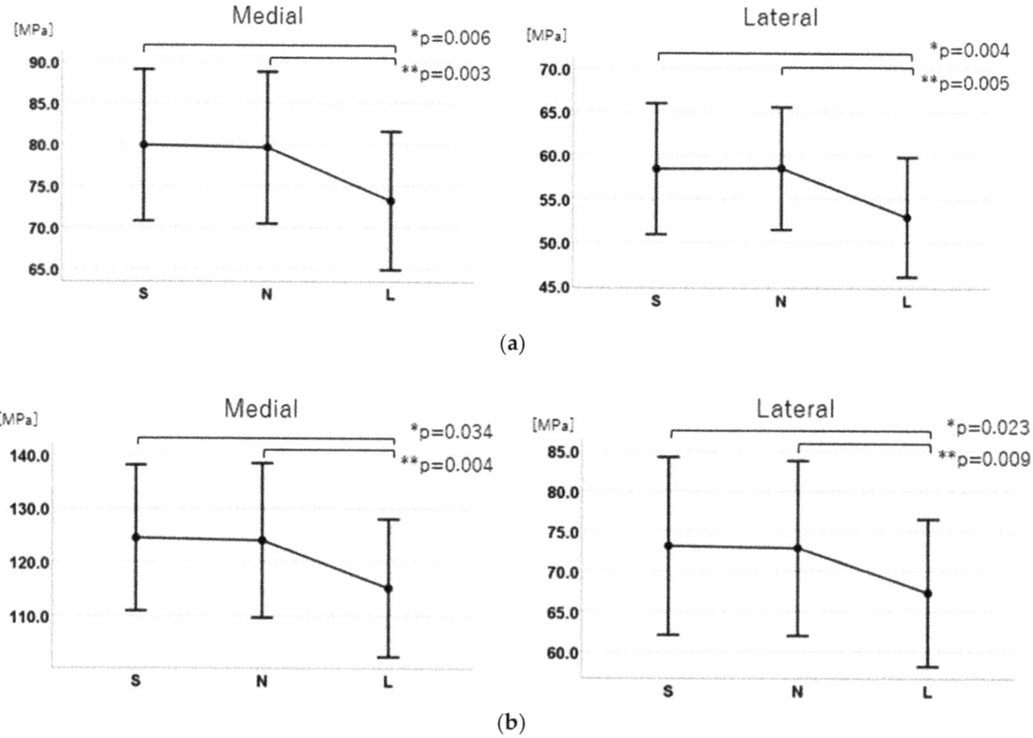

Figure 9. Comparison of the maximum equivalent stress values. (**a**) Normal walking; (**b**) Stair climbing. In both the normal walking and stair-climbing conditions, a significant difference was observed between Groups S and L (*), as well as between Groups N and L (**). However, no significant difference was found between Groups S and N.

3.5.2. Stair Climbing

a. Comparison between groups

For the medial side, the stress was 124.5 (95% CI: 110.84–138.06) MPa for the S group, 124.0 (95% CI: 109.6–138.4) MPa for the N group, and 115.1 (95% CI: 102.3–128.0) MPa for the L group. For the lateral side, it was 73.1 (95% CI: 62.1–84.2) MPa for the S group, 72.9 (95% CI: 62.0–83.8) MPa for the N group, and 67.3 (95% CI: 58.2–76.5) MPa for the L group. Both medial and lateral sides showed significant main effects in the analysis of variance (medial side: $F(2, 58) = 7.220$, $p = 0.004$, $\eta^2 = 0.20$; lateral side: $F(2, 58) = 6.110$, $p = 0.004$, $\eta^2 = 0.17$) (Figure 9).

b. Post-hoc multiple comparisons

Significant differences were found between the S and L groups and the N and L groups on both the medial and lateral sides (S vs. L: medial, $p = 0.034$; lateral, $p = 0.023$; N vs. L, medial $p = 0.004$, lateral $p = 0.009$). On the medial side, the S group showed 9.30 MPa higher stress than the L group (95% CI: 0.55–18.06) and 8.87 MPa higher stress than the N group (95% CI: 2.59–15.15). On the lateral side, the S group had 5.81 MPa higher stress than the L group (95% CI: 0.64–10.98) and 5.56 MPa higher stress than the N group (95% CI: 1.18–9.93). No significant differences were found between the S and N groups (medial and lateral: $p > 0.99$) (Figure 9).

4. Discussion

Simulations were performed using the FEA cTHA model, showing that the average equivalent stress at the distal screw removal hole decreased as the stem length increased. The maximum equivalent stress at the distal screw removal hole showed significant differences between the S and L groups, as well as between the N and L groups, but no significant difference was found between the S and N groups. This is the first study to investigate in detail the impact of stem length on stress distribution around the distal screw removal hole in cTHA using FEA and statistical analysis.

Several studies have examined the relationship between cortical bone defects and bone strength using biomechanical techniques. In cadaver experiments, circular defects less than 20–30% of bone diameter had no significant effect on torsional strength [51,52]. Animal studies, such as those by Edgerton et al. on sheep femurs, showed no significant decrease in torsional strength with 10% defects, whereas 20% defects led to a 34% decrease, and a linear decrease in strength was observed with up to 60% defects [53]. Ho et al. found a 38% reduction in energy absorption with a 4-mm cortical defect in pig femurs [54]. Howieson et al. reported a 47% reduction in energy absorption with three 3.5-mm cortical defects in calves [55], and Brooks et al. showed a 55.2% reduction in energy absorption with 2.8-mm or 3.6-mm drill holes in dog femurs [56]. These studies suggest that following intramedullary nail removal, a 5-mm screw extraction hole in the femoral shaft may significantly reduce energy absorption, but its effect on torsional strength might not be as large.

The cortical bone defect should be bridged with a stem length at least twice the diameter of the femur (approximately 40 mm) [39–41]. Clinically, similar treatment strategies are often employed for stem-type fractures, such as Vancouver types B2 and B3, where the fracture site is bridged [40,41,57,58]. Several studies have biomechanically verified the bridging of cortical bone defects in femurs associated with cTHA, primarily reporting on the nail-plate fixation concept, where it was found that fracture did not occur even without a large stem bridging over screw extraction holes [33] and that a stem length of 1.5 × the femur diameter minimized stresses at the screw extraction site in cadaver experiments [59].

For continuous circumferential cortical defects such as fractures, sufficient strength, rigidity, and axial stability must be obtained via stem bridging. As previously mentioned, a bridging length that is at least twice the femoral diameter is recommended. However, for partial and smaller cortical bone defects such as those from implant removal holes, the impact on bone strength is limited, and the level of strength and stability required for fracture treatment is not necessary. The purpose of bridging in cTHA is to reinforce strength and rigidity against vulnerability from cortical bone defects and to reduce stress, and the required bridging length may be shorter than that for fractures or larger cortical bone defects.

Currently, a wide variety of stems and techniques are used in cTHA. However, no clinically significant method has been identified, and stem selection is largely at the surgeon's discretion [7,11,34,35,37,38,60–63]. Furthermore, there are concerns regarding cement leakage and BCIS exist in cemented stems [61]. Several measures have been reported to prevent cement leakage, such as using gloves inflated with saline, bone wax, bone plugs made from the femoral head, and reinserting screws [33,64]. Generally, cement use is considered suitable for relatively older adult patients aged >70 years, especially in environments that are not conducive to osseointegration, such as poor bone quality or wide medullary cavities [8,34,63,65,66]. In contrast, many orthopedic surgeons prefer cementless stems, which provide more physiologically and biologically favorable fixation while avoiding cement leakage and BCIS [11,34,35,67]. Many surgeons use long stems to bridge screw extraction holes [11,34,35,37]. Good outcomes with cementless stems coated with hydroxyapatite over the entire circumference have also been reported in cTHA [57].

Structurally vulnerable areas such as screw extraction holes are prone to stress concentration, which increases the risk of fracture. Using a stem of insufficient length positioned close to the screw extraction site may lead to a hinge effect around this area, causing stress concentration. However, the insertion of a sufficiently long stem can distribute the load across a wide region of the femur. Because of its increased rigidity, this stem reduces the stress around the screw extraction hole by transferring the stress along the stem. The stem also potentially reinforces structural integrity around this weak point.

In this study, the distal screw length (femur diameter) averaged 25.7 $\pm$ 1.7 mm, with a screw diameter of 5 mm, equating to an approximately 20% bicortical bone defect. Based on biomechanical studies, this defect size may significantly reduce energy absorption, making it essential to bridge the distal screw extraction hole with a sufficiently long stem to reduce stress and prevent fractures.

In this study, the short stem (120 mm) overlapped the distal screw extraction hole, whereas the normal (130 mm) and long (160 mm) stems were bridged by approximately 10 mm and 40 mm, respectively. Bridging of 10 mm was insufficient to avoid stress concentration, whereas bridging of 40 mm (approximately 1.6 times the femoral cortex diameter) significantly reduced peak stress around the extraction hole. Therefore, the optimal stem length to reduce the maximum stress around the distal screw extraction hole is likely to be between 130 and 160 mm.

While long stems in cTHA have been associated with increased operative time, blood loss, and perioperative complications compared to standard stems [68], it is ideal to use a stem that meets the required bridging length. However, owing to the limited available stem options, revision of long stems may be necessary in practice. Special attention is required to prevent intraoperative fractures, and careful handling is required during surgery.

This study used FEA to simulate different stem lengths in cTHA models, providing a detailed analysis of the stress around the distal screw extraction hole, which has not been well understood previously. FEA allows stress measurement within the extraction hole, which is a challenge for traditional methods such as strain gauges or thermoelastic stress analysis. Additionally, using existing patient CT data, we reduced costs and ensured a sufficient sample size for statistical analysis. This enabled us to determine the stem length required to reduce the peak stress on the screw extraction hole.

Given that cortical bone defects may serve as points for stress accumulation, we believe that the observed significant reduction in maximum stress around screw holes with the use of a 160 mm long stem could have important clinical implications, thereby elevating the risk of fractures [8]. Specifically, it may contribute to mitigating the risk of screw hole-related fractures, which represent a notable concern in cTHA.

This study also has some limitations. First, this study was conducted under ideal conditions with bone and boundary conditions that differed from those in vivo. Specifically, the bone microstructure and dynamic load conditions were not fully represented in the model. We used MF software (version 13.0), which estimates bone density from CT values and allows FEA to incorporate the bone microstructure.

The static loading model in FEA has inherent limitations that restrict its ability to fully replicate real-world conditions. It fails to account for dynamic factors, such as time-dependent loading during activities like walking or impact, limiting its relevance for fatigue or vibration analysis. The simplification of boundary conditions often neglects the complex interactions between implants, bones, and surrounding tissues, reducing the model's physiological accuracy. Nonlinear behaviors, including plastic deformation, friction, or material detachment, are frequently omitted, which can compromise the reliability of results in high-stress regions. Additionally, static models are constrained to single loading conditions, making them inadequate for evaluating cyclic loads or fatigue behavior over time.

Crucially, static models do not incorporate biological responses, such as bone remodeling or adaptation around implants, which are essential for long-term outcome predictions. While effective for assessing stress and deformation under specific conditions, static loading models require supplementary dynamic or fatigue analyses to capture the complexity of real-world biomechanical environments.

CT scanners play a critical role in determining the accuracy of FEA models. Higher-resolution scans not only capture precise geometric details and density distributions of bone, enhancing model fidelity but also increase data volume and computational cost. Lower resolutions, while more efficient, risk oversimplifying key structural features.

HU is vital for defining material properties, allowing the incorporation of bone density and regional variations. However, artifacts, particularly from metal implants, can introduce errors and require effective image processing for correction. Scan resolution also impacts mesh generation. Excessively fine meshes derived from high-resolution data can reduce computational efficiency, making it essential to balance detail and performance through appropriate simplifications tailored to the purpose of analysis. High-resolution scans are indispensable for analyzing intricate bone structures, while lower resolutions may suffice for broader stress distribution evaluations. Understanding and optimizing CT scanner settings based on analytical objectives is key to achieving accurate and efficient results.

Additionally, we modeled the highest load levels during daily activities based on previous studies, accounting for soft tissue dynamics to approximate real-life scenarios. Second, fracture lines, calluses formation, and bone sclerosis around the screw removal site were not included to simplify the model, which can lead to potentially underestimating the localized stress distribution and structural weakness. Building a model based on femur CT data after intramedullary nail insertion could represent fracture lines, callus formation, and sclerosis. However, metal artifacts complicate accurate CT value detection and stress analysis. Therefore, post-nail removal CT data are preferred, although cases involving only nail removal and subsequent CT scans are rare. Consequently, we reconstructed a nail extraction model by aligning 3D femur models with intramedullary nail STL data and substituting the nail's physical properties with an "unused material" designation in MF. Third, we focused solely on stem length without considering width (canal fill ratio), shape, or fixation concepts. The selected #11 stem may not ideally match each patient's medullary canal shape, although we controlled for the canal shape using the Dorr classification to select samples with similar canal morphology.

This study suggests that a sufficient bridging length for the screw extraction hole lies between 10 and 40 mm and recommends the use of long stems in cTHA following intramedullary nail surgeries. Future directions include further verification with 20 mm and 30 mm bridging lengths to determine the optimal bridging length. Additional studies using cemented stems for Dorr type B and C, as well as experimental and clinical trials, are needed to validate the FEA results with fracture strength testing.

5. Conclusions

In cTHA following intramedullary nailing for femoral trochanteric fractures, using a sufficiently long stem may reduce the stress concentration around the distal screw extraction holes, potentially lowering the risk of periprosthetic fractures. Selecting an appropriate stem length is crucial to minimize the risk of complications associated with cTHA.

Author Contributions: Conceptualization, K.S.; methodology, K.S.; software, K.S. and R.W.; validation, K.S.; formal analysis, K.S.; investigation, K.S., F.H., and S.Y.; resource, K.S., T.Y., R.W., F.H., and S.Y.; data curation, K.S., F.H., and S.Y.; writing-original draft preparation, K.S.; writing-review and editing, T.N., T.Y., R.W., and H.M.; visualization, K.S.; supervision, T.N., T.Y., R.W., and H.M.; project administration, T.N., T.Y., R.W., and H.M. All authors have read and agreed to the published version of the manuscript.

Funding: This research received no external funding.

Institutional Review Board Statement: This retrospective study was approved by the Ethics Committee of the University of Tsukuba Hospital, approval code: H27-041 on 14 August 2022.

Informed Consent Statement: Informed consent was obtained from all subjects involved in the study.

Data Availability Statement: The data are available from the corresponding author if required.

Acknowledgments: The authors would like to thank Teijin Nakashima Medical (Okayama, Japan) for providing the STL data of the Universia stem.

Conflicts of Interest: The authors declare no conflicts of interest.

References

1. Hip Fracture: Management. Available online: https://www.ncbi.nlm.nih.gov/books/NBK553768/ (accessed on 23 November 2024).
2. O'Connor, M.I.; Switzer, J.A. AAOS Clinical Practice Guideline Summary: Management of hip fractures in older adults. *J. Am. Acad. Orthop. Surg.* **2022**, *30*, e1291–e1296. [CrossRef] [PubMed]
3. Geller, J.A.; Saifi, C.; Morrison, T.A.; Macaulay, W. Tip-apex distance of intramedullary devices as a predictor of cut-out failure in the treatment of peritrochanteric elderly hip fractures. *Int. Orthop.* **2010**, *34*, 719–722. [CrossRef] [PubMed]
4. Mavrogenis, A.F.; Panagopoulos, G.N.; Megaloikonomos, P.D.; Igoumenou, V.G.; Galanopoulos, I.; Vottis, C.T.; Karabinas, P.; Koulouvaris, P.; Kontogeorgakos, V.A.; Vlamis, J.; et al. Complications after hip nailing for fractures. *Orthopedics* **2016**, *39*, e108–e116. [CrossRef] [PubMed]
5. Mokka, J.; Kirjasuo, K.; Koivisto, M.; Virolainen, P.; Junnila, M.; Seppänen, M.; Äärimaa, V.; Isotalo, K.; Mäkelä, K.T. Hip arthroplasty after failed nailing of proximal femoral fractures. *Eur. J. Orthop. Surg. Traumatol.* **2012**, *3*, 231–237. [CrossRef]
6. Murena, L.; Moretti, A.; Meo, F.; Saggioro, E.; Barbati, G.; Ratti, C.; Canton, G. Predictors of cut-out after cephalomedullary nail fixation of pertrochanteric fractures: A retrospective study of 813 patients. *Arch. Orthop. Trauma. Surg.* **2018**, *138*, 351–359. [CrossRef]
7. DeHaan, A.M.; Groat, T.; Priddy, M.; Ellis, T.J.; Duwelius, P.J.; Friess, D.M.; Mirza, A.J. Salvage hip arthroplasty after failed fixation of proximal femur fractures. *J. Arthroplasty* **2013**, *28*, 855–859. [CrossRef]
8. Haidukewych, G.J.; Berry, D.J. Hip arthroplasty for salvage of failed treatment of intertrochanteric hip fractures. *J. Bone Joint Surg. Am.* **2003**, *85*, 899–904. [CrossRef]

9. Hammad, A.; Abdel-Aal, A.; Said, H.G.; Bakr, H. Total hip arthroplasty following failure of dynamic hip screw fixation of fractures of the proximal femur. *Acta Orthop. Belg.* **2008**, *74*, 788–792.
10. Sharvill, R.J.; Ferran, N.A.; Jones, H.G.; Jones, S.A. Long-stem revision prosthesis for salvage of failed fixation of extracapsular proximal femoral fractures. *Acta Orthop. Belg.* **2009**, *75*, 340–345.
11. Shi, X.; Zhou, Z.; Yang, J.; Shen, B.; Kang, P.; Pei, F. Total hip arthroplasty using non-modular cementless long-stem distal fixation for salvage of failed internal fixation of intertrochanteric fracture. *J. Arthroplasty* **2015**, *30*, 1999–2003. [CrossRef]
12. Exaltacion, J.J.F.; Incavo, S.J.; Mathews, V.; Parsley, B.; Noble, P. Hip arthroplasty after intramedullary hip screw fixation: A perioperative evaluation. *J. Orthop. Trauma.* **2012**, *26*, 141–147. [CrossRef] [PubMed]
13. Corró, S.; Óleo-Taltavull, R.; Teixidor-Serra, J.; Tomàs-Hernández, J.; Selga-Marsà, J.; García-Sánchez, Y.; Guerra-Farfán, E.; Andrés-Peiró, J.-V. Salvage hip replacement after cut-out failure of cephalomedullary nail fixation for proximal femur fractures: A case series describing the technique and results. *Int. Orthop.* **2022**, *46*, 2775–2783. [CrossRef] [PubMed]
14. Archibeck, M.J.; Carothers, J.T.; Tripuraneni, K.R.; White, R.E., Jr. Total hip arthroplasty after failed internal fixation of proximal femoral fractures. *J. Arthroplasty* **2013**, *28*, 168–171. [CrossRef] [PubMed]
15. Winemaker, M.; Gamble, P.; Petruccelli, D.; Kaspar, S.; de Beer, J. Short-term outcomes of total hip arthroplasty after complications of open reduction internal fixation for hip fracture. *J. Arthroplasty* **2006**, *21*, 682–688. [CrossRef]
16. Haentjens, P.; Casteleyn, P.P.; Opdecam, P. Hip arthroplasty for failed internal fixation of intertrochanteric and subtrochanteric fractures in the elderly patient. *Arch. Orthop. Trauma. Surg.* **1994**, *113*, 222–227. [CrossRef]
17. Douglas, S.J.; Remily, E.A.; Sax, O.C.; Pervaiz, S.S.; Delanois, R.E.; Johnson, A.J. How does conversion total hip arthroplasty compare to primary? *J. Arthroplasty* **2021**, *36*, S155–S159. [CrossRef]
18. Solarino, G.; Bizzoca, D.; Dramisino, P.; Vicenti, G.; Moretti, L.; Moretti, B.; Piazzolla, A. Total hip arthroplasty following the failure of intertrochanteric nailing: First implant or salvage surgery? *World J. Orthop.* **2023**, *14*, 763–770. [CrossRef]
19. Tetsunaga, T.; Fujiwara, K.; Endo, H.; Noda, T.; Tetsunaga, T.; Sato, T.; Shiota, N.; Ozaki, T. Total hip arthroplasty after failed treatment of proximal femur fracture. *Arch. Orthop. Trauma. Surg.* **2017**, *137*, 417–424. [CrossRef]
20. Gjertsen, J.E.; Lie, S.A.; Fevang, J.M.; Havelin, L.I.; Engesaeter, L.B.; Vinje, T.; Furnes, O. Total hip replacement after femoral neck fractures in elderly patients: Results of 8,577 fractures reported to the Norwegian Arthroplasty Register. *Acta Orthop.* **2007**, *78*, 491–497. [CrossRef]
21. Mortazavi, S.M.; M, R.G.; Bican, O.; Kane, P.; Parvizi, J.; Hozack, W.J. Total hip arthroplasty after prior surgical treatment of hip fracture is it always challenging? *J. Arthroplasty* **2012**, *27*, 31–36. [CrossRef]
22. Abdel, M.P.; Watts, C.D.; Houdek, M.T.; Lewallen, D.G.; Berry, D.J. Epidemiology of periprosthetic fracture of the femur in 32 644 primary total hip arthroplasties: A 40-year experience. *Bone Joint J.* **2016**, *98-B*, 461–467. [CrossRef]
23. Ashkenazi, I.; Amzallag, N.; Factor, S.; Abadi, M.; Morgan, S.; Gold, A.; Snir, N.; Warschawski, Y. Age as a risk factor for intraoperative periprosthetic femoral fractures in cementless hip hemiarthroplasty for femoral neck fractures: A retrospective analysis. *Clin. Orthop. Surg.* **2024**, *16*, 41–48. [CrossRef] [PubMed]
24. Morice, A.; Ducellier, F.; Bizot, P. Total hip arthroplasty after failed fixation of a proximal femur fracture: Analysis of 59 cases of intra- and extra-capsular fractures. *Orthop. Traumatol. Surg. Res.* **2018**, *104*, 681–686. [CrossRef]
25. Berry, D.J. Periprosthetic fractures associated with osteolysis: A problem on the rise. *J. Arthroplasty* **2003**, *18*, 107–111. [CrossRef]
26. Puri, S.; Sculco, P.K.; Abdel, M.P.; Wellman, D.S.; Gausden, E.B. Total hip arthroplasty after proximal femoral nailing: Preoperative preparation and intraoperative surgical techniques. *Arthroplast. Today* **2023**, *24*, 101243. [CrossRef] [PubMed]
27. Chen, D.W.; Lin, C.L.; Hu, C.C.; Tsai, M.F.; Lee, M.S. Biomechanical consideration of total hip arthroplasty following failed fixation of femoral intertrochanteric fractures—A finite element analysis. *Med. Eng. Phys.* **2013**, *35*, 569–575. [CrossRef]
28. Beals, R.K.; Tower, S.S. Periprosthetic fractures of the femur. An analysis of 93 fractures. *Clin. Orthop. Relat. Res.* **1996**, *327*, 238–246. [CrossRef]
29. Lindahl, H.; Garellick, G.; Regnér, H.; Herberts, P.; Malchau, H. Three hundred and twenty-one periprosthetic femoral fractures. *J. Bone Joint Surg. Am.* **2006**, *88*, 1215–1222. [CrossRef]
30. Morishima, T.; Ginsel, B.L.; Choy, G.G.H.; Wilson, L.J.; Whitehouse, S.L.; Crawford, R.W. Periprosthetic Fracture Torque for Short Versus Standard Cemented Hip Stems: An Experimental In Vitro Study. *J. Arthroplasty* **2014**, *29*, 1067–1071. [CrossRef]
31. Bishop, N.E.; Burton, A.; Maheson, M.; Morlock, M.M. Biomechanics of Short Hip Endoprostheses—The Risk of Bone Failure Increases with Decreasing Implant Size. *Clin. Biomech.* **2010**, *25*, 666–674. [CrossRef]
32. Jakubowitz, E.; Seeger, J.B.; Lee, C.; Heisel, C.; Kretzer, J.P.; Thomsen, M.N. Do Short-Stemmed Prostheses Induce Periprosthetic Fractures Earlier than Standard Hip Stems? A Biomechanical Ex-Vivo Study of Two Different Stem Designs. *Arch. Orthop. Trauma. Surg.* **2009**, *129*, 849–855. [CrossRef] [PubMed]
33. Zhang, B.; Chiu, K.Y.; Wang, M. Hip arthroplasty for failed internal fixation of intertrochanteric fractures. *J. Arthroplasty* **2004**, *19*, 329–333. [CrossRef] [PubMed]

34. Moon, N.H.; Shin, W.C.; Kim, J.S.; Woo, S.H.; Son, S.M.; Suh, K.T. Cementless total hip arthroplasty following failed internal fixation for femoral neck and intertrochanteric fractures: A comparative study with 3-13 years' follow-up of 96 consecutive patients. *Injury* **2019**, *50*, 713–719. [CrossRef] [PubMed]
35. Thakur, R.R.; Deshmukh, A.J.; Goyal, A.; Ranawat, A.S.; Rasquinha, V.J.; Rodriguez, J.A. Management of failed trochanteric fracture fixation with cementless modular hip arthroplasty using a distally fixing stem. *J. Arthroplasty* **2011**, *26*, 398–403. [CrossRef]
36. Patterson, B.M.; Salvati, E.A.; Huo, M.H. Total hip arthroplasty for complications of intertrochanteric fracture. A technical note. *J. Bone Joint Surg. Am.* **1990**, *72*, 776–777. [CrossRef]
37. D'Arrigo, C.; Perugia, D.; Carcangiu, A.; Monaco, E.; Speranza, A.; Ferretti, A. Hip arthroplasty for failed treatment of proximal femoral fractures. *Int. Orthop.* **2010**, *34*, 939–942. [CrossRef]
38. Yuan, B.J.; Abdel, M.P.; Cross, W.W.; Berry, D.J. Hip arthroplasty after surgical treatment of intertrochanteric hip fractures. *J. Arthroplasty* **2017**, *32*, 3438–3444. [CrossRef]
39. Dennis, D.A.; Dingman, C.A.; Meglan, D.A.; O'Leary, J.F.; Mallory, T.H.; Berme, N. Femoral cement removal in revision total hip arthroplasty. A biomechanical analysis. *Clin. Orthop. Relat. Res.* **1987**, *220*, 142–147. [CrossRef]
40. Larson, J.E.; Chao, E.Y.; Fitzgerald, R.H. Bypassing femoral cortical defects with cemented intramedullary stems. *J. Orthop. Res.* **1991**, *9*, 414–421. [CrossRef]
41. Klein, A.H.; Rubash, H.E. Femoral windows in revision total hip arthroplasty. *Clin. Orthop. Relat. Res.* **1993**, *291*, 164–170. [CrossRef]
42. Dorr, L.D.; Faugere, M.C.; Mackel, A.M.; Gruen, T.A.; Bognar, B.; Malluche, H.H. Structural and cellular assessment of bone quality of proximal femur. *Bone* **1993**, *14*, 231–242. [CrossRef] [PubMed]
43. UNIVERSIA STEM. Available online: https://formedic.teijin-nakashima.co.jp/products/detail/?id=524 (accessed on 23 December 2024).
44. Hirata, Y.; Inaba, Y.; Kobayashi, N.; Ike, H.; Fujimaki, H.; Saito, T. Comparison of mechanical stress and change in bone mineral density between two types of femoral implant using finite element analysis. *J. Arthroplasty* **2013**, *28*, 1731–1735. [CrossRef] [PubMed]
45. Tano, A.; Oh, Y.; Fukushima, K.; Kurosa, Y.; Wakabayashi, Y.; Fujita, K.; Yoshii, T.; Okawa, A. Potential bone fragility of mid-shaft atypical femoral fracture: Biomechanical analysis by a CT-based nonlinear finite element method. *Injury* **2019**, *50*, 1876–1882. [CrossRef] [PubMed]
46. Keyak, J.H.; Rossi, S.A.; Jones, K.A.; Skinner, H.B. Prediction of femoral fracture load using automated finite element modeling. *J. Biomech.* **1998**, *31*, 125–133. [CrossRef] [PubMed]
47. Bergmann, G.; Bender, A.; Dymke, J.; Duda, G.; Damm, P. Standardized loads acting in hip implants. *PLoS ONE* **2016**, *11*, e0155612. [CrossRef]
48. Heller, M.O.; Bergmann, G.; Kassi, J.P.; Claes, L.; Haas, N.P.; Duda, G.N. Determination of muscle loading at the hip joint for use in pre-clinical testing. *J. Biomech.* **2005**, *38*, 1155–1163. [CrossRef]
49. Biemond, J.E.; Aquarius, R.; Verdonschot, N.; Buma, P. Frictional and bone ingrowth properties of engineered surface topographies produced by electron beam technology. *Arch. Orthop. Trauma. Surg.* **2011**, *131*, 711–718. [CrossRef]
50. Noble, P.C.; Alexander, J.W.; Lindahl, L.J.; Yew, D.T.; Granberry, W.M.; Tullos, H.S. The anatomic basis of femoral component design. *Clin. Orthop. Relat. Res.* **1988**, *235*, 148–165. [CrossRef]
51. Minear, W.L.; Tachdjian, M.O. Hip dislocation in cerebral palsy. *J. Bone Joint Surg. Am.* **1956**, *38*, 1358–1364.
52. Burstein, A.H.; Currey, J.; Frankel, V.H.; Heiple, K.G.; Lunseth, P.; Vessely, J.C. Bone strength. The effect of screw holes. *J. Bone Joint Surg. Am.* **1972**, *54*, 1143–1156. [CrossRef]
53. Edgerton, B.C.; An, K.N.; Morrey, B.F. Torsional strength reduction due to cortical defects in bone. *J. Orthop. Res.* **1990**, *8*, 851–855. [CrossRef] [PubMed]
54. Ho, K.W.; Gilbody, J.; Jameson, T.; Miles, A.W. The effect of 4 mm bicortical drill hole defect on bone strength in a pig femur model. *Arch. Orthop. Trauma. Surg.* **2010**, *130*, 797–802. [CrossRef] [PubMed]
55. Howieson, A.J.; Jones, M.D.; Theobald, P.S. The change in energy absorbed post removal of metalwork in a simulated paediatric long bone fracture. *J. Child. Orthop.* **2014**, *8*, 443–447. [CrossRef]
56. Brooks, D.B.; Burstein, A.H.; Frankel, V.H. The biomechanics of torsional fractures. The stress concentration effect of a drill hole. *J. Bone Joint Surg. Am.* **1970**, *52*, 507–514. [CrossRef]
57. Springer, B.D.; Berry, D.J.; Lewallen, D.G. Treatment of periprosthetic femoral fractures following total hip arthroplasty with femoral component revision. *J. Bone Joint Surg. Am.* **2003**, *85*, 2156–2162. [CrossRef]
58. Mulay, S.; Hassan, T.; Birtwistle, S.; Power, R. Management of types B2 and B3 femoral periprosthetic fractures by a tapered, fluted, and distally fixed stem. *J. Arthroplasty* **2005**, *20*, 751–756. [CrossRef]
59. Panjabi, M.M.; Trumble, T.; Hult, J.E.; Southwick, W.O. Effect of femoral stem length on stress raisers associated with revision hip arthroplasty. *J. Orthop. Res.* **1985**, *3*, 447–455. [CrossRef]

60. Lee, Y.-K.; Kim, J.T.; Alkitaini, A.A.; Kim, K.-C.; Ha, Y.-C.; Koo, K.-H. Conversion hip arthroplasty in failed fixation of intertrochanteric fracture: A propensity score matching study. *J. Arthroplasty* **2017**, *32*, 1593–1598. [CrossRef]
61. Mahmoud, S.S.; Pearse, E.O.; Smith, T.O.; Hing, C.B. Outcomes of total hip arthroplasty, as a salvage procedure, following failed internal fixation of intracapsular fractures of the femoral neck: A systematic review and meta-analysis. *Bone Joint J.* **2016**, *98*, 452–460. [CrossRef]
62. Angelini, M.; McKee, M.D.; Waddell, J.P.; Haidukewych, G.; Schemitsch, E.H. Salvage of failed hip fracture fixation. *J. Orthop. Trauma.* **2009**, *23*, 471–478. [CrossRef]
63. Zeng, X.; Zhan, K.; Zhang, L.; Zeng, D.; Yu, W.; Zhang, X.; Zhao, M. Conversion to total hip arthroplasty after failed proximal femoral nail antirotations or dynamic hip screw fixations for stable intertrochanteric femur fractures: A retrospective study with a minimum follow-up of 3 years. *BMC Musculoskelet. Disord.* **2017**, *18*, 38. [CrossRef] [PubMed]
64. Langdown, A.J.; Low, A.K.; Auld, J.W.; Bruce, W.J.; Walker, P.M. Technique for preventing cement extrusion from screw holes during conversion of failed hip fracture fixation to total hip replacement. *Ann. R. Coll. Surg. Engl.* **2005**, *87*, 473–474. [PubMed]
65. Müller, F.; Galler, M.; Zellner, M.; Bäuml, C.; Füchtmeier, B. Total hip arthroplasty after failed osteosynthesis of proximal femoral fractures: Revision and mortality of 80 patients. *J. Orthop. Surg.* **2017**, *25*, 2309499017717869. [CrossRef] [PubMed]
66. Hsu, C.J.; Chou, W.Y.; Chiou, C.P.; Chang, W.N.; Wong, C.Y. Hemi-arthroplasty with supplemental fixation of greater trochanter to treat failed hip screws of femoral intertrochanteric fracture. *Arch. Orthop. Trauma. Surg.* **2008**, *128*, 841–845. [CrossRef]
67. Laffosse, J.M.; Molinier, F.; Tricoire, J.L.; Bonnevialle, N.; Chiron, P.; Puget, J. Cementless modular hip arthroplasty as a salvage operation for failed internal fixation of trochanteric fractures in elderly patients. *Acta Orthop. Belg.* **2007**, *73*, 729–736.
68. Shi, T.; Fang, X.; Huang, C.; Li, W.; You, R.; Wang, X.; Xia, C.; Zhang, W. Conversion hip arthroplasty using standard and long stems after failed internal fixation of intertrochanteric fractures. *Orthop. Surg.* **2023**, *15*, 124–132. [CrossRef]

Journal of
Clinical Medicine

MDPI

Article

Enhancing Stability of Pediatric Femoral Fractures Treated with Elastic Nail Using an External Fixator

Barak Rinat [1,*], Eytan Dujovny [1], Noam Bor [1,2], Nimrod Rozen [1,2], Avi Chezar [1] and Guy Rubin [1,2]

1 Orthopedic Department, Emek Medical Center, Afula 1834111, Israel; eytan.dujovny1@gmail.com (E.D.); noambor@yahoo.com (N.B.); chezarmd@gmail.com (A.C.); guyrubinmd@gmail.com (G.R.)
2 Faculty of Medicine, Technion, Haifa 3525433, Israel
* Correspondence: barakrinat@gmail.com; Tel.: +972-54-8120046; Fax: +972-4-6494201

Abstract: Background: Diaphyseal femoral fractures in children older than 5 years and before adolescence are usually treated surgically. The literature describes several surgical techniques; however, we present an additional minimally invasive technique that combines the use of elastic intramedullary nails and a uniplanar external fixator as an optional solution for managing more complex cases. **Method**: This was a retrospective review of four children aged 9–12 years who suffered from unstable diaphyseal femoral fractures and were admitted to our institution. **Results**: We treated four children between the years 2021 and 2023. All patients underwent closed reduction of their fractures and fixation with an elastic intramedullary nail and an external fixator. Full radiographic fracture healing with acceptable alignment was achieved in all patients. The minimum clinical follow-up was 1.5 years. No major complications were observed, and all patients achieved full clinical recovery as well as proper limb alignment and length. **Conclusions**: Fixation of complex diaphyseal femoral fractures using a combination of internal and external fixation is a simple technique that avoids the need for extensive soft tissue exposure while also promoting fracture stability and maintenance of bone length and rotation. This method can be incorporated into the armamentarium of orthopedic surgeons as an additional solution for addressing more challenging cases.

Keywords: diaphyseal femur fracture; elastic intramedullary nails; external fixation; pediatric

1. Introduction

Diaphyseal femoral fractures require submuscular plating, as fracture malunion and other surgical complications appear to be more prevalent. The fracture pattern, that is, whether the fracture is considered stable or unstable, is another important consideration. Stable diaphyseal fractures with transverse or short oblique patterns are relatively common injuries in the pediatric population, with a reported incidence of approximately 20 per 100,000 [1–3]. The accepted treatment for preschool children below 5 years of age is most commonly nonsurgical with spica casting, either immediately or after a few days of in-hospital skin traction [4]; for patients nearing the end of growth and beyond, adult-type surgical techniques of rigid intramedullary nailing are the common treatment. For patients aged 5–12 years, several treatment options may be considered without clear guidelines or strict treatment strategies; however, surgical treatment is generally mandatory.

The two most common fixation techniques are elastic intramedullary nailing (ESIN) and submuscular plating, with patient weight and fracture pattern being the two significant parameters influencing the surgeon's decision. Heavy body weight (>50 kg) usually mandates a more rigid fixation; as such, non-obese patients are commonly treated with

ESIN [5]. Conversely, unstable fractures, such as long, oblique, spiral, or comminuted, or fractures at the edges of the diaphysis, such as subtrochanteric and distal diaphyseal, are commonly treated with submuscular plating [6–12]. Each technique has disadvantages; residual angular malalignment and limb length discrepancy are attributed more to ESIN, whereas soft tissue damage and more extensile surgical exposure are attributed to submuscular plate fixation.

A third emerging option, more relevant to the upper part of this age group, involves the use of rigid intramedullary nailing, similar to adult intramedullary nailing. Limitations for the younger portion of this group include a small medullary canal diameter and potential harm to the trochanteric apophysis. Piriformis-fossa entry rigid nails were used in the past to avoid growth plate injuries but are less popular nowadays because of the risk of damaging the femoral head blood supply. Pediatric-adjusted lateral trochanteric entry points have become popular, with promising results regarding the potential risk of trochanteric growth arrest [13].

A fourth surgical option, the use of external fixation, is reserved for the deployed environment, damage control treatment, or severe soft tissue compromise and is usually a bridging solution before a definitive one [14,15]. Lastly, fewer documented surgical options were described by Anderson et al. in 2017 [16]. They described a combined method using both ESIN and an external fixator for unstable pediatric femoral fractures in two patients. However, only one of the two cases described was treated primarily with this method, whereas the second patient was treated with the combined method because of surgical complications after primary plate fixation. We present four additional cases of preadolescent children aged 9–12 years who sustained femoral diaphyseal fractures that were unstable or had severe soft tissue compromise and whose primary and definitive surgical treatment was combined with both ESIN and a uniplanar external fixator.

2. Patients and Methods

Publication of this paper was approved by the local IRB (institutional review board). Four patients aged 9–12 years who were operated on and followed postoperatively at our pediatric orthopedic unit between 2021 and 2023, were included in the study. All children were admitted to the hospital with isolated thigh trauma, underwent emergency care clearance, and were diagnosed with a diaphyseal femoral fracture with no additional concomitant injuries (Table 1).

Table 1. Characteristics of pediatric patients with diaphyseal femoral fractures treated with ESINs and an external fixator.

No.	Age (Years)	Gender	Side	Fracture Pattern	Cause	Surgical Technique	Removal of Ex-Fix (Months)	Removal of ESINs (Months)	Complications
1	9.8	Male	R	Mid-diaphyseal long spiral	Direct hit	Retrograde ESINs and uniplanar Ex-Fix	1.5	7	Pin-tract infection
2	10.3	Female	L	Distal diaphyseal long spiral	Fall	Retrograde ESINs and uniplanar Ex-Fix	3	17	Irritable ESIN LLD 0.5cm

Table 1. *Cont.*

No.	Age (Years)	Gender	Side	Fracture Pattern	Cause	Surgical Technique	Removal of Ex-Fix (Months)	Removal of ESINs (Months)	Complications
3	12.5	Male	L	Comminuted subtrochanteric	Fall	Retrograde ESINs and uniplanar Ex-Fix	2	14	Irritable ESIN
4	12.5	Male	R	Butterfly, subtrochanteric	Fall from horse	Retrograde ESINs and uniplanar Ex-Fix	1.8	n/a	none

The publication of the current paper was approved by the local institutional review board. Four patients, three boys and one girl aged 9–12 years, who were operated on and followed postoperatively at our pediatric orthopedic unit between the years 2021 and 2023, were included in the study. All children were initially admitted to the hospital emergency unit with isolated thigh trauma, underwent primary emergency care clearance, and were diagnosed with a diaphyseal femoral fracture with no additional concomitant injuries (Table 1).

Surgical Technique

All patients were evaluated preoperatively and, owing to the characteristics of their fractures, were operated on using the combined technique of ESIN and a uniplanar external fixator as a primary surgical technique. All surgeries were performed by the same senior pediatric orthopedic surgical team. Following a satisfactory temporary closed reduction, two 3.5 mm elastic intramedullary nails (Titanium Elastic Nail (TEN), DePuy Synthes, Oberdorf, Switzerland) were inserted in an antegrade fashion from the distal metaphyseal femur, medially and laterally, through the fracture and proximally up to the trochanteric region.

Owing to the fractures' unstable patterns, two to four 6 mm hydroxyapatite-coated Schanz pins (OsteoTite pins, Orthofix, Lewisville, TX, USA) were implanted laterally, with one or two on each end of the fracture, and connected with a uniplanar external fixator (Orthofix Limb Reconstruction System (LRS), Orthofix, Lewisville, TX, USA) (Figures 1a and 2a,b).

All patients received a non-weight-bearing regimen and were routinely followed up at our pediatric orthopedic outpatient clinic. Six to 12 weeks postoperatively, when satisfactory radiological healing was observed, the patient was admitted, and the external fixator was removed under general anesthesia (Figure 1b,c). Full weight-bearing with intense physiotherapy was initiated instantly. The patients were clinically and radiographically followed in a pediatric orthopedic clinic by the same team for a minimum of 12 months.

The four patients included in this study were evaluated preoperatively by the same pediatric orthopedic surgeons, and owing to the characteristics of their fractures and their age and weight, they were operated on using the combined technique of elastic intramedullary nails and a uniplanar external fixator as the primary surgical technique. All four surgeries were performed by the same senior pediatric orthopedic surgical team. Following a satisfactory temporary closed reduction under fluoroscopy, two 3.5 mm elastic intramedullary nails (Titanium Elastic Nail (TEN), DePuy Synthes, USA) were inserted in a retrograde fashion from the distal metaphyseal femur medially and laterally, using minimal incisions, through the fracture site, and proximally up to the trochanteric region.

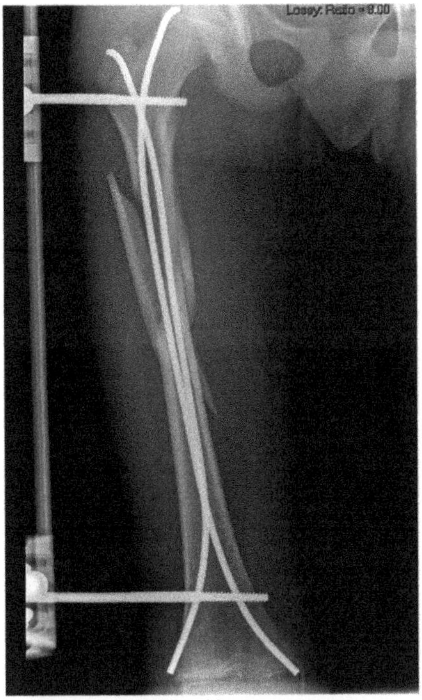

(**a**)

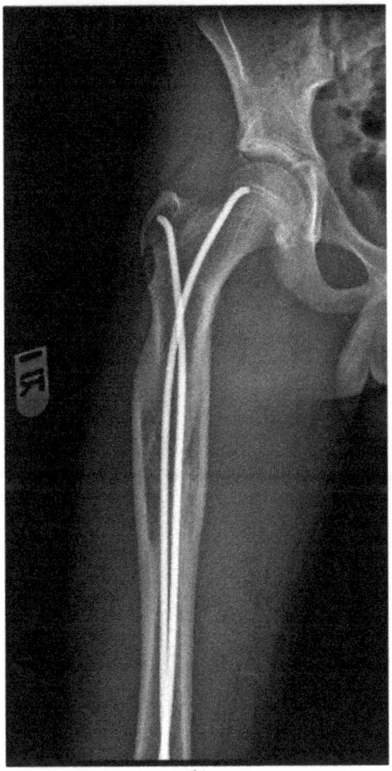

(**b**)

Figure 1. *Cont.*

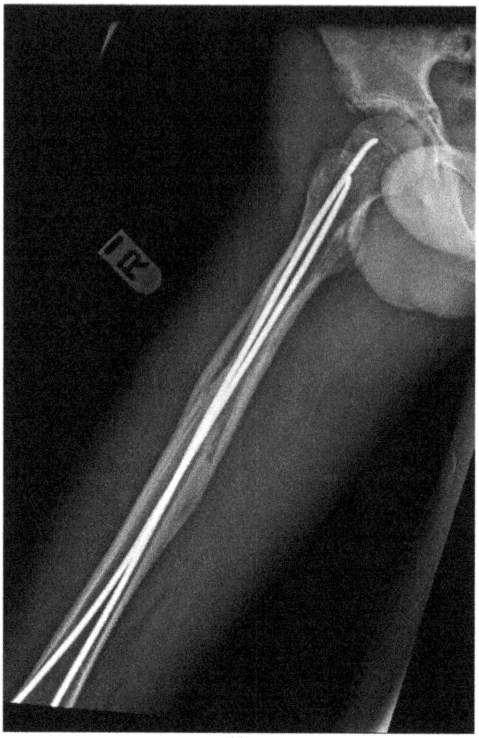

(c)

Figure 1. A 12-year-old male with a butterfly subtrochanteric fracture. (**a**) Immediate postoperative radiograph. (**b**,**c**) Twelve-week postoperative radiographs, anteroposterior and lateral views.

Owing to the fractures' unstable patterns, which were demonstrated both before and after operation, further torsional stability and length control were needed; therefore, two or four 6 mm hydroxyapatite-coated Schanz pins (OsteoTite pins, Orthofix, USA) were implanted from the lateral side of the femur through minimal incisions. Each Schanz pin was carefully inserted with accurate perpendicular bicortical fixation, with one or two pins on each end of the fracture. The pins were inserted at a posterior position to the elastic nails to prevent any contact between the external device and the internal fixation. Finally, all the Schanz pins were connected together with a uniplanar external fixator (Orthofix Limb Reconstruction System (LRS), Orthofix, USA) (Figures 1a and 2a,b).

Postoperatively, all patients received a non-weight-bearing regimen with meticulous physiotherapy and were routinely followed up at our pediatric orthopedic outpatient clinic. Six to twelve weeks postoperatively, when satisfactory radiological healing was observed, the patient was admitted to the hospital and the external fixator was removed under general anesthesia (Figure 1b,c). Full weightbearing with further intense physiotherapy was initiated instantly. The patients were clinically and radiographically followed in a pediatric orthopedic clinic by the same team for a minimum of 12 months.

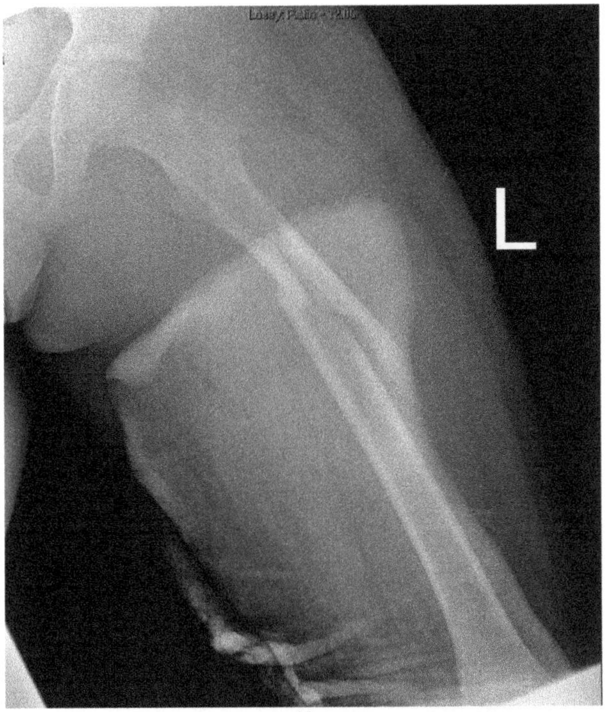

(a)

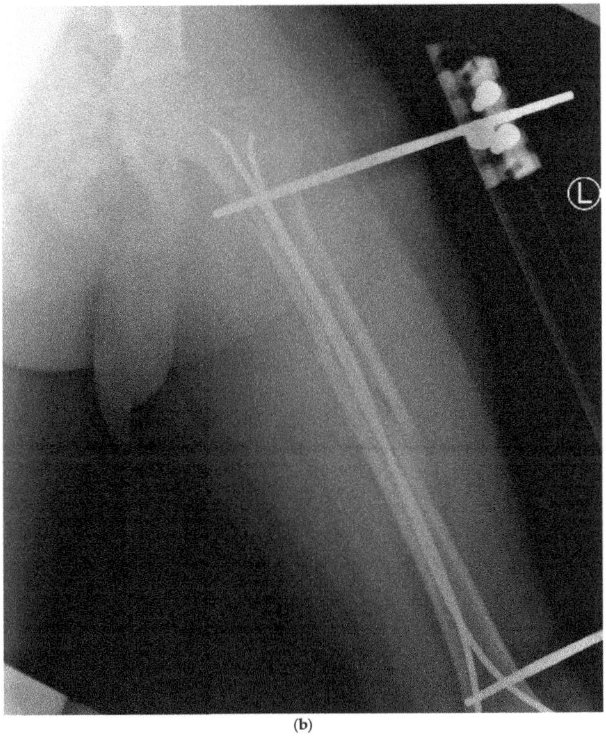

(b)

Figure 2. *Cont.*

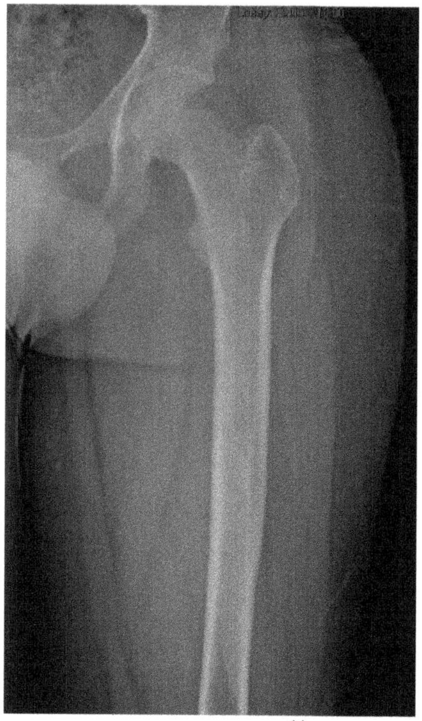

(c)

Figure 2. A 12.5-year-old with a subtrochanteric fracture with extension into the proximal femur. (**a**) Emergency room radiograph demonstrating a left subtrochanteric fracture with proximal extension. (**b**) Immediate postoperative radiograph with the uniplanar external fixator and two elastic intramedullary nails (ESINs). (**c**) After removal of the ESINs, with full fracture healing.

3. Results

None of the four patients in our case series had any major surgical or injury-related complications, including refracture, deep infection, vascular injury, neurologic deficits, or chronic pain. Two patients experienced knee stiffness prior to the removal of the external fixator, but following the physiotherapy regimen, both gained full range of motion within a few months. One patient was diagnosed with a pin-tract infection a few days before the six-week postoperative follow-up. Foul odor with cloudy discharge from the pin wounds warranted the admittance of the patient to the orthopedic department, and the external fixator was removed. The infection resolved following a week of intravenous antibiotics followed by oral antibiotics. Two patients who were symptomatic due to prominent ESINs proximal to the knee joints at the distal thigh, had them removed under general anesthesia 14 months postoperatively (Figure 1c). All patients regained a fully symmetrical range of motion of the hip and knee joints. No patient had a clinically significant limb length discrepancy or angular deformity.

4. Discussion

Treating femoral fractures in the pediatric population can be challenging. Due to the high bone remodeling potential at preschool age, nonoperative solutions are acceptable or even recommended, while at older ages, nonunion, residual axial deformity, rotational deformity, or limb-length discrepancy are worrisome complications that often mandate surgery [17,18].

The choice of technical solution varies according to the patient's age, body weight, and fracture pattern. However, no significant overall advantage has been shown regarding the chosen method [19], and each method has benefits and disadvantages. Narayanan et al. [20] demonstrated that femoral fracture fixation with intramedullary elastic nails alone, although technically relatively simple with minimal soft tissue and bone exposure, has relatively high complication rates, with up to 50% of prominent symptomatic nail edges, and a high rate of malunion, with approximately 12% of patients requiring reoperation prior to union. For comminuted fractures, which are unstable, the group recommends stricter post-operative follow-up and further immobilization. Submuscular plating for unstable pediatric femoral fractures seems to have fewer complications than ESIN [21] but requires a longer operative time for both the initial fixation and the removal of the plate [9]. In fractures where submuscular plates are implanted, a second surgery is recommended, especially if the implant is relatively distal. Although the removal of the plate can be time-consuming and technically more challenging with relatively extensile soft tissue exposure, the retention of submuscular plates may result in angular deformities, leg-length discrepancies, or prominent hardware [22].

In our case series, we described an alternative for the primary treatment of the more complex femoral diaphyseal fractures, using a combined surgical technique of both elastic intramedullary nails and a uniplanar external fixator, in a fashion similar to that previously described in one of two cases by Anderson et al. [16]. The advantage of using an external fixator for femoral fracture reduction has been previously described by our group [23]; however, in the current technique, the fixator, beyond being a temporary assisting tool for reduction and rotational control, is also part of the final fracture fixation. In our opinion, in correctly selected cases of preadolescent complex unstable or comminuted diaphyseal femoral fractures, this technique is appropriate and allows for minimal surgical exposure, minimal blood loss, no soft tissue stripping, and relatively affordable and more importantly available hardware. In a biomechanical study by Wilton et al. [24], the augmentation of elastic nails with an external fixator demonstrated excellent stability and rotational control, potentially eliminating some of the main disadvantages of ESIN alone [24]. Early and technically simple removal of the external fixator permits good rehabilitation and decreases the risk of infection while maintaining the elastic nails facilitates additional stability until full healing is observed.

However, we acknowledge that the disadvantages of this technique should be considered. The need for at least one additional general anesthesia for external fixator removal and the risk of pin tract infection are not negligible considerations. Careful insertion of the implants without any direct contact is important to reduce the risk of intramedullary infection. Nonetheless, on the basis of our experience, we believe that this technique should be part of the pediatric orthopedic trauma surgeon armamentarium for treating diaphyseal femoral fractures, as it provides more versatility in treatment options, especially in more challenging cases of pediatric preadolescent femoral fractures.

5. Conclusions

Complex unstable diaphyseal fractures in the preadolescent population poses a technical challenge for the treating surgeon. At this age, there are several surgical solutions, each with benefits and weaknesses. We hope that the combined method described in our study of fracture fixation using an external fixator with elastic intramedullary nails adds a substantially useful tool that expands the number of available surgical solutions and offers yet another appropriate treatment option.

Author Contributions: Conceptualization, B.R.; Methodology, E.D. and G.R.; Validation, A.C.; Formal analysis, B.R.; Investigation, E.D. and N.B.; Writing—review & editing, B.R.; Supervision, A.C., N.R. and G.R. All authors have read and agreed to the published version of the manuscript.

Funding: This research received no external funding.

Institutional Review Board Statement: The study was conducted according to the guidelines of the Declaration of Helsinki, and approved by the local IRB (Institutional review board) of Haemek Medical Center (protocol code 0185-16-EMC and 8 January 2017).

Informed Consent Statement: Patient consent was waived due to retrospective study.

Data Availability Statement: The raw data supporting the conclusions of this article will be made available by the authors on request.

Conflicts of Interest: The authors declare no conflict of interest.

References

1. Hinton, R.Y.; Lincoln, A.; Crockett, M.M.; Sponseller, P.; Smith, G. Fractures of the femoral shaft in children. Incidence, mechanisms, and sociodemographic risk factors. *J. Bone Jt. Surg Am.* **1999**, *81*, 500–509. [CrossRef]
2. Engström, Z.; Wolf, O.; Hailer, Y.D. Epidemiology of pediatric femur fractures in children: The Swedish Fracture Register. *BMC Musculoskelet. Disord.* **2020**, *21*, 796. [CrossRef] [PubMed]
3. von Heideken, J.; Svensson, T.; Blomqvist, P.; Haglund-Åkerlind, Y.; Janarv, P.M. Incidence and Trends in Femur Shaft Fractures in Swedish Children Between 1987 and 2005. *J. Pediatr. Orthop.* **2011**, *31*, 512–519. [CrossRef] [PubMed]
4. Ramo, B.A.; Martus, J.E.; Tareen, N.; Hooe, B.S.; Snoddy, M.C.; Jo, C.H. Intramedullary Nailing Compared with Spica Casts for Isolated Femoral Fractures in Four and Five-Year-Old Children. *J. Bone Jt. Surg. Am.* **2016**, *98*, 267–275. [CrossRef]
5. Ho, C.A.; Skaggs, D.L.; Tang, C.W.; Kay, R.M. Use of flexible intramedullary nails in pediatric femur fractures. *J. Pediatr. Orthop.* **2006**, *26*, 497–504. [CrossRef] [PubMed]
6. Shaha, J.; Cage, J.M.; Black, S.; Wimberly, R.L.; Shaha, S.H.; Riccio, A.I. Flexible Intramedullary Nails for Femur Fractures in Pediatric Patients Heavier Than 100 Pounds. *J. Pediatr. Orthop.* **2018**, *38*, 88–93. [CrossRef]
7. Donovan, R.L.; Harries, L.; Whitehouse, M.R. Flexible nails have a significantly increased risk of complications compared with plating techniques when treating diaphyseal femoral fractures in children aged 5-12: A systematic review. *Injury* **2020**, *51*, 2763–2770. [CrossRef] [PubMed]
8. Li, Y.; Hedequist, D.J. Submuscular plating of pediatric femur fracture. *J. Am. Acad. Orthop. Surg.* **2012**, *20*, 596–603. [CrossRef] [PubMed]
9. Chen, L.K.; Sullivan, B.T.; Sponseller, P.D. Submuscular plates *versus* flexible nails in preadolescent diaphyseal femur fractures. *J. Child. Orthop.* **2018**, *12*, 488–492. [CrossRef]
10. Wilson, C.H.; Smith, C.S.; Gay, D.M.; Loveless, E.A. Submuscular locked plating of pediatric femur fractures. *J. Surg. Orthop. Adv.* **2012**, *21*, 136–140. [CrossRef] [PubMed]
11. Samora, W.P.; Guerriero, M.; Willis, L.; Klingele, K.E. Submuscular Bridge Plating for Length-Unstable, Pediatric Femur Fractures. *J. Pediatr. Orthop.* **2013**, *33*, 797–802. [CrossRef]
12. Kanlic, E.M.; Anglen, J.O.; Smith, D.G.; Morgan, S.J.; Pesántez, R.F. Advantages of Submuscular Bridge Plating for Complex Pediatric Femur Fractures. *Clin. Orthop. Relat. Res.* **2004**, *426*, 244–251. [CrossRef]
13. Keeler, K.A.; Dart, B.; Luhmann, S.J.; Schoenecker, P.L.; Ortman, M.R.; Dobbs, M.B.; Gordon, J.E. Antegrade intramedullary nailing of pediatric femoral fractures using an interlocking pediatric femoral nail and a lateral trochanteric entry point. *J. Pediatr. Orthop.* **2009**, *29*, 345–351. [CrossRef]
14. Eichinger, J.K.; McKenzie, C.S.; Devine, J.G. Evaluation of pediatric lower extremity fractures managed with external fixation: Outcomes in a deployed environment. *Am. J. Orthop.* **2012**, *41*, 15–19. [PubMed]
15. Bar-On, E.; Sagiv, S.; Porat, S. External fixation or flexible intramedullary nailing for femoral shaft fractures in children. A prospective, randomised study. *J. Bone Jt. Surg. Br.* **1997**, *79*, 975–978. [CrossRef]
16. Anderson, S.R.; Nelson, S.C.; Morrison, M.J. Unstable Pediatric Femur Fractures: Combined Intramedullary Flexible Nails and External Fixation. *J. Orthop. Case Rep.* **2017**, *7*, 32–35. [PubMed]
17. Kocher, M.S.; Sink, E.L.; Blasier, R.D.; Luhmann, S.J.; Mehlman, C.T.; Scher, D.M.; Matheney, T.; Sanders, J.O.; Watters, W.C., 3rd; Goldberg, M.J.; et al. Treatment of pediatric diaphyseal femur fractures. *J. Am. Acad. Orthop. Surg.* **2009**, *17*, 718–725. [CrossRef]
18. Anglen, J.O.; Choi, L. Treatment options in pediatric femoral shaft fractures. *J. Orthop. Trauma* **2005**, *19*, 724–733. [CrossRef] [PubMed]

19. Flynn, J.M.; Schwend, R.M. Management of pediatric femoral shaft fractures. *J. Am. Acad. Orthop. Surg.* **2004**, *12*, 347–359. [CrossRef]
20. Narayanan, U.G.; Hyman, J.E.; Wainwright, A.M.; Rang, M.; Alman, B.A. Complications of Elastic Stable Intramedullary Nail Fixation of Pediatric Femoral Fractures, and How to Avoid Them. *J. Pediatr. Orthop.* **2004**, *24*, 363–369. [CrossRef]
21. May, C.; Yen, Y.M.; Nasreddine, A.Y.; Hedequist, D.; Hresko, M.T.; Heyworth, B.E. Complications of plate fixation of femoral shaft fractures in children and adolescents. *J. Child. Orthop.* **2013**, *7*, 235–243. [CrossRef]
22. Kelly, B.; Heyworth, B.; Yen, Y.M.; Hedequist, D. Adverse sequelae due to plate retention following submuscular plating for pediatric femur fractures. *J. Orthop. Trauma* **2013**, *27*, 726–729. [CrossRef]
23. Bor, N.; Rozen, N.; Dujovny, E.; Rubin, G. Fixator-Assisted Plating in Pediatric Supracondylar Femur Fractures. *Glob. Pediatr. Health* **2019**, *6*, 1–5. [CrossRef] [PubMed]
24. Wilton, P.J.; Burke, C.A.; Inceoglu, S.; Nelson, S.C.; Morrison, M.J. External fixator-augmented flexible intramedullary nailing of an unstable pediatric femoral shaft fracture model: A biomechanical study. *J. Pediatr. Orthop. B* **2020**, *29*, 485–489. [CrossRef] [PubMed]

Journal of
Clinical Medicine

MDPI

Technical Note

Continuous Compression Implants in Foot and Ankle Surgery: Tips and Tricks

Konstantinos Tsikopoulos [1,*], Konstantinos Sidiropoulos [2], Dimitrios Kitridis [3], Constantinos Loizou [4] and Alisdair Felstead [5]

1 Orthopaedic Department, North Bristol NHS Trust, Bristol BS10 5NB, UK
2 Orthopaedic Department, Florina General Hospital, 531 00 Florina, Greece; kcdroq@yahoo.gr
3 Orthopaedic Department, 424 General Military Hospital, 564 29 Thessaloniki, Greece; dkitridis@gmail.com
4 Orthopaedic Department, Oxford University Hospitals NHS Trust, Oxford OX3 9DU, UK; constantinos.loizou@ouh.nhs.uk
5 Orthopaedic Department, Portsmouth Hospitals NHS Trust, Portsmouth PO6 3FT, UK; alisdair.felstead@porthosp.nhs.uk
* Correspondence: kostastsikop@gmail.com

Abstract: Background: Continuous Compression Implants (CCIs) are low-profile implants made of nitinol and titanium. They offer multiple benefits in comparison to plate and screw fixation for foot and ankle indications, and they are designed in such a way that they continuously and dynamically compress the opposed bony surfaces throughout the entire healing process. **Methods:** In this study, we present our experience on the use of those nitinol implants for midfoot and hindfoot surgery. Furthermore, we elaborate on the advantages and downsides of using this internal fixation method and highlight common pitfalls which could lead to undesirable clinical outcomes. We also demonstrate our proposed surgical technique on how to use CCIs in a reproducible and reliable way and present surgical tips which could help reduce surgical time when utilising these implants. We also make surgical recommendations on their use and present the underlying biomechanics, which could provide a better understanding of the rationale behind using them in the field of foot and ankle surgery. Last but not least, we presented the early clinical and radiological results of a series of patients who underwent primary midfoot fusion for Lisfranc injury between 2020 and 2023. **Results:** With a minimum follow-up of 9 months, satisfactory clinical and radiological union was noted in all those patients. The mean difference between pre- and post-operative MOxFQ scores was −37.7 (95% CI was 16.9 to 58.5; $p = 0.03$). The mean post-operative VAS pain at rest was 3.2 (SD = 2.3). No major complications were noted. **Conclusions:** CCI internal fixation is a safe, reproducible, and reliable method when it comes to foot and ankle conditions, but it requires appropriate pre-operative planning, surgical training, and careful implantation.

Keywords: continuous compression implants; staples; midfoot/hindfoot fusion; Lisfranc; surgical technique

1. Introduction

Definition

Nitinol Continuous Compression Implants (CCIs) are low-profile implants manufactured from nitinol and titanium (approximately at a 50/50% ratio). They feature pseudo-elastic properties and shape-memory in addition to good corrosion resistance, no cytotoxic, genotoxic, or allergic activity, and excellent biocompatibility [1]. The word "ni-ti-nol" is derived from the metals utilised, that is, nickel and titanium, in addition to "nol", which stands for Naval Ordnance Laboratory, as the U.S. military first utilised this biomaterial in 1965 along with W.J. Buehler. CCIs are designed in such a way that they continuously and dynamically compress the opposed bony surfaces throughout the entire healing process [1]. The ultimate goal of utilising these implants is to minimise the effects of bone resorption and maintain a stable construct. Also, another rationale is to recover compression after repetitive loading.

From an evolutionary standpoint, static staples were first utilised, and they were made of stainless steel or titanium. They only provided minimal compression (if any), and they were prone to distal gapping. Subsequently, the first nitinol staples were body temperature-activated, and they required freezer storage and heating prior to activation. On the contrary, the new-generation super-elastic nitinol compression staples are ready to use at room temperature, and no activation is needed.

It is worthy of note that CCIs could potentially be advantageous over traditional fixation methods since they enable smaller surgical incisions, decrease surgical time compared to plate and screw fixation, provide continuous compression that leads to satisfactory union rates post-operatively, and cause less irritation in the midfoot/hindfoot area where there is limited overlying soft tissue due to their low profile [2]. Nevertheless, we wish to highlight that the continuous compression forces provided by the CCIs cannot compensate for inappropriate joint preparation when it comes to midfoot/hindfoot fusions.

When compared to other established methods of fusion fixation, such as the crossed-screw and plate-and-screw techniques, comparable biomechanical performance has been documented [1,3]. In more detail, nitinol staples demonstrate increased compression surface area and the improved recovery of plantar gaping after mechanical loading when compared to plate-and-screw constructs [4,5]. Moreover, an activated Nitinol implant self-adjusts over time to continuously and dynamically compress together the opposing bony surfaces. To elaborate further, the implant initially comes in a closed position, which provides secure fixation and resists migration, with the bowing bridge allowing for the even distribution of the compression forces along the near and far cortices. Consequently, when the implant is loaded in an open position, the compression forces are stored similar to a powerful spring. During the implantation phase, the implant is released in bone, which in turn allows for dynamic compression as the staple attempts to return to its initial closed design shape. It should be noted that CCIs come at a relatively high cost compared to plate and screw fixation, and therefore, the accurate placement of the implants is recommended as they can only be deployed once.

2. Materials and Methods

Institutional review board approval was obtained, and the data utilised in this paper were retrospectively collected to review the efficacy and complications following fusion surgery for foot and ankle indications. The Elite BME (Synthes USA, LLC, Monument, CO, USA; or Bio-Medical Enterprises, Inc., San Antonio, TX, USA) and SpeedTitan continuous compression staples (Synthes USA, LLC, Monument, CO, USA; or Bio-Medical Enterprises, Inc., San Antonio, TX, USA) were used in a single institution by two fellowship-trained foot and ankle surgeons between 2021 and 2023. Inclusion criteria were patients between the ages of 18 and 85 years of age requiring fusion for foot and ankle conditions such as midfoot/hindfoot arthrosis and acquired flat foot deformity. We excluded diabetic patients and advanced osteoporosis. A subset of patients requiring Lisfranc fusion was further analysed from a clinical and radiological point of view. The primary outcome was the clinical and radiological union. The secondary outcomes included the assessment of functional disability as measured with the Manchester–Oxford Foot Questionnaire

(MOxFQ), pain at rest as expressed with a visual analogue scale (VAS), and post-operative complications. The included patients were randomly selected from the local hospital database using computerised software. For the case series on Lisfranc fusions presented in this paper, 41 patients were assessed for eligibility, and 6 of those were considered in the analysis. A minimum of 9 months follow-up was considered.

For the midfoot fusions presented in this paper, early clinical and radiological results were evaluated. The primary outcome was the clinical and radiological union. The secondary outcomes included the assessment of functional disability as measured with the Manchester–Oxford Foot Questionnaire (MOxFQ), pain at rest as expressed with a visual analogue scale (VAS) at rest, and post-operative complications. The statistical analysis was performed with the SPSS software (Version 27.0. Armonk, NY, USA: IBM Corp.) and a p value of 0.05 indicated statistical significance.

2.1. Surgical Technique

For the joint preparation, a combination of chisels, osteotomes, and curettes was utilised. This was followed by the appropriate fenestration of the subchondral plate with drill bits, and bone grafting was utilised as required at that stage.

We highlight that the 'perfect circle technique' was implemented prior to introducing the implants to avoid undesirable joint penetration, which would inevitably compromise the compression across the fusion site and result in pain and patient dissatisfaction. This 'perfect circle technique' involved the use of the staple guide along with the corresponding staple guidewires. This construct was then screened with the image intensifier, and the radiograph was considered satisfactory when the holes on either side of the staple guide were perfectly superimposed (Figure 1).

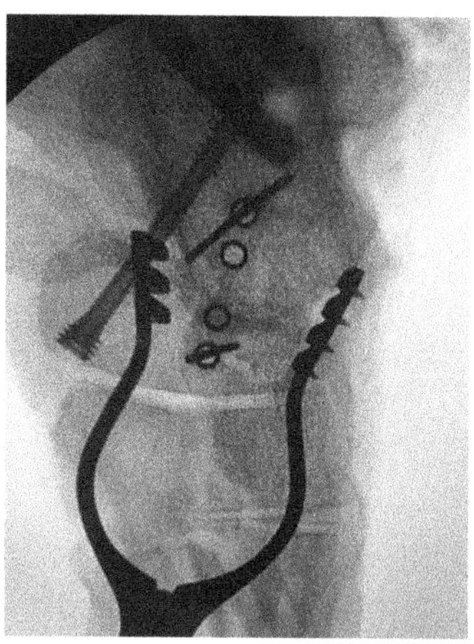

Figure 1. Intra-operative image of talonavicular joint fusion demonstrating the 'perfect circle technique'.

This translates to an image of a round circle in the guide rather than an ellipse. To quickly achieve perfect circles without specific instrumentation, the surgeon should manipulate the position of the foot in relation to the drill guide, which remains in place throughout the wire and subsequent pin placement. Moreover, a true lateral view is highly recommended for the surgeon to confirm that the position of the wires is not intra-articular. To effectively prevent this complication from happening, the surgeon should be mindful of the orientation of the joints (e.g., saddle-shaped calcaneocuboid joint).

2.2. Results Following Primary Fusion for Lisfranc Injuries

We retrospectively identified 6 adult patients (mean age and BMI were 46 years and 33.4 kg/m^2, respectively) who underwent primary fusion for their midfoot injuries between 2020 and 2023. With a minimum follow-up of 9 months, satisfactory clinical and radiological union was noted in all patients. The mean difference between pre- and post-operative MOxFQ scores was −37.7 (95% CI was 16.9 to 58.5; $p = 0.03$). The mean post-operative VAS pain at rest was 3.2 (SD = 2.3). No major complications were noted.

3. Discussion

3.1. Recommendations on the Arm Length, Number of Staples per Joint, and Number of Legs Are Given Below

Regarding the ideal length of the arms, evidence has shown that the CCIs enable compression distal to their tip (Figure 2).

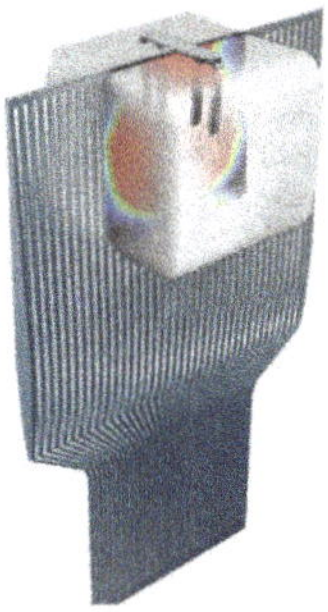

Figure 2. Illustration depicting the compression area, which expands beyond the tip of the continuous compression staple based on biomechanical measurements.

Therefore, we advocate that it is safe to use shorter arms than the depth of the bone, particularly when there is a high risk of breaching the adjacent joint, thus causing irritation. In more detail, in terms of the ideal length of the legs, biomechanical evidence has shown that the bicortical placement of nitinol staples is not required to achieve adequate compression. To elaborate further, the same amount of compression can be achieved when placing staples 2 mm short of the far cortex when compared with bicortical placement. Moreover, from a biomechanical point of view, troughing does not appear to affect the properties of the construct. Therefore, the intentional troughing of the bone during implant placement will result not only in less implant prominence but also in no changes to the biomechanical properties/compression capacity of the nitinol staples [6]. In addition, we wish to highlight the fact that although no clear guidelines on the ideal length of the staples exist, evidence has shown that a 20 mm bridge length exhibits higher contact forces and lower stresses as compared to 15 mm bridge length, thus suggesting that the longer the bridge length, the more stable the internal fixation [7].

At present, there are no published guidelines as to how many staples should be used per joint, despite the fact that biomechanical studies have shown that two staples provide a biomechanically sound construct featuring increased stiffness, joint contact area, and peak load [4]. In our experience, compression can be assessed intra-operatively following the introduction of the CCIs, and depending on the subsequent visual and radiographic assessment performed by the surgeon, a further implant could be considered.

In terms of the legs of the staples, there are no clear recommendations in the literature at the moment. From a biomechanical perspective, where possible, four-leg staples should be utilised to allow for the even distribution of compression forces through the tips. For instance, this could be the case for the first tarsometatarsal joint [2] (Figure 3). Of note, dual-staple constructs applied in an orthogonal fashion provide greater than doubled compression in comparison to constructs with a single staple. Moreover, double-staple constructs appear to be 2 times stiffer than plate constructs. This finding may have potential implications in clinical practice as double-staple constructs should be used where feasible [5].

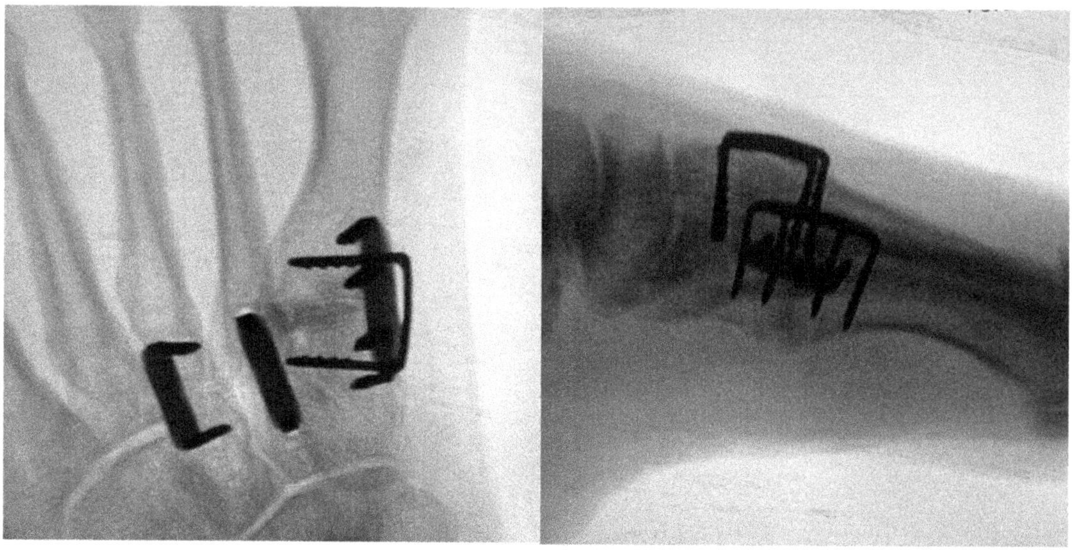

Figure 3. Intra-operative radiographs depicting fusion of tarsometatarsal joints with a combination of two- and four-leg staples.

3.2. Assessment of Union Post-Operatively

For a fusion to be considered radiologically successful, a minimum of 50% healing is required [8]. On top of that, broken hardware is suggestive of a nonunion. From a clinical standpoint, continued pain/discomfort in the subsequent clinic follow-ups denotes clinical nonunion. If in doubt 9 months post-operatively, a CT scan is warranted.

From a radiological standpoint, the majority of studies utilise plain radiography as the main imaging modality when it comes to evaluating the union rates following fusion with continuous compression staples. It is worthy of note that although CT features higher sensitivity and specificity for union detection, only a limited number of authors have implemented it in their papers [9,10].

At this point, we wish to draw the readers' attention to the fact that a "disguise" nonunion may be seen in patients rarely. This phenomenon occurs when radiographs do not depict the nonunion, given the continuous compression exerted by the continuous compression staples [11]. In other words, one of the downsides of using CCIs could be that nonunion may appear radiographically occult on plain radiographs.

3.3. Broken Metalwork and Requirement for Hardware Removal

Of note, staples with a narrow bridge carry a higher risk of fatigue failure as their bending stiffness appears to be insufficient when it comes to midfoot and hindfoot fusions (Figure 4).

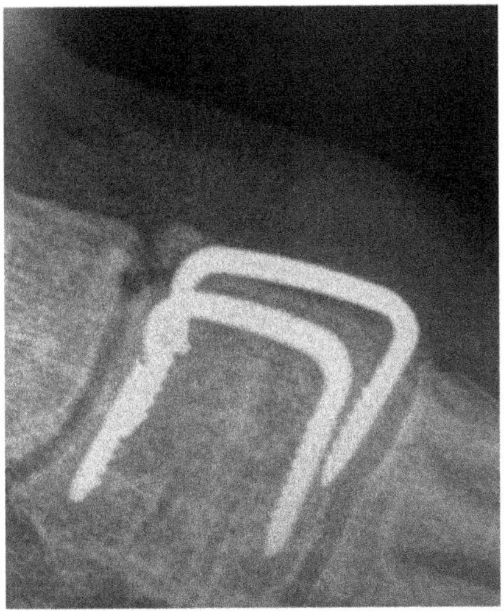

Figure 4. Lateral midfoot radiograph depicting broken metalwork 6 months following tarsometatarsal joint fusion.

The incidence of nonunion in the presence of broken nitinol staples appears to be high [12]. In terms of the removal of hardware due to secondary pain, it appears that the plate-and-screw constructs present a higher rate in comparison to the staple-only construct [13].

3.4. Factors Affecting Biomechanical Performance/Risk Factors for Nonunion

It is undeniable that results following internal fixation with nitinol staples are influenced by the bone quality [14]. Moreover, further risk factors for union include a BMI equal to or greater than 35, the fusion of the Chopart joints (especially in isolation), surgery for diabetic patients, and male patients. Therefore, utilising nitinol staples in isolation in osteoporotic bones is not recommended, and caution should be exercised when considering the application of bone grafting.

3.5. Examples of CCI Application for Foot and Ankle Indications

CCIs can be effectively used either alone or in conjunction with other fixation methods (e.g., plates and screws). Moreover, they can be used not only for fusions but also for securing extra-articular osteotomies (e.g., distal metatarsal, Akin, Evans, Cotton).

In our experience, we have found CCIs particularly useful in the setting of a triple fusion as the tourniquet time is of the essence (Figure 5). In more detail, we claim that CCIs could result in less peroneal tendon irritation when compared to plates for a calcaneocuboid fusion. Regarding the talonavicular joint, recent evidence has demonstrated that CCIs exhibit equivalent functional/biomechanical properties when compared to the "gold standard" lag screws [15]. In a recent systematic review with a total of nine articles looking at talonavicular arthrodesis, fusion rates were found to be higher in the staple fixation group (i.e., 100%, n = 13) than in the screw fixation one (n = 75)—87.5% to 100% [16].

Likewise, based on our experience, we highly recommend the use of CCIs for midfoot fusions, such as naviculocuneiform and tarsometatarsal joints, as irritation from metalwork is less likely compared to plate and screw fixation (Figure 6).

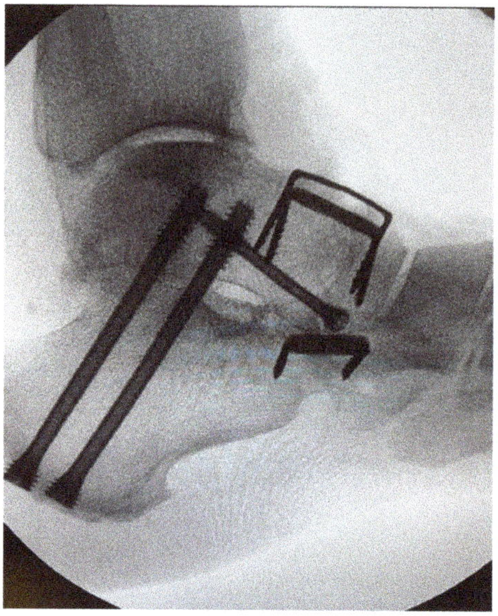

Figure 5. Lateral intra-operative radiograph depicting a realignment triple fusion performed with a combination of internal fixation techniques including CCIs. Note that the dorsal osteophytes at the talonavicular joint were debrided to allow for appropriate staple position, thus preventing anterior ankle impingement.

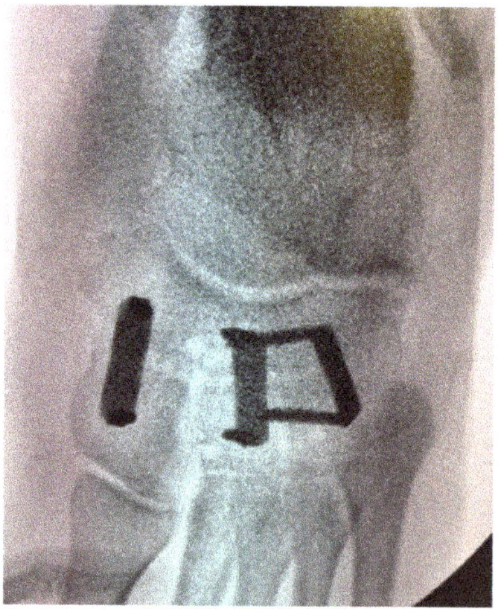

Figure 6. Intra-operative anteroposterior radiograph depicting a naviculocuneiform joint fusion with CCI fixation.

Regarding the first tarsometatarsal joint, multiple studies have demonstrated that the efficacy of CCIs is satisfactory, with a fusion rate of approximately 90% and a patient satisfaction rate similar to that seen with other fixation methods [17]. In our experience, the 90-90-degree configuration technique yields satisfactory outcomes and essentially requires placement of two staples, one in the dorsal and the second in the medial position (Figure 7). Of note, those two staples should be sequentially tamped down to the bone to ensure that the arms would not interfere with each other, thus compromising compression.

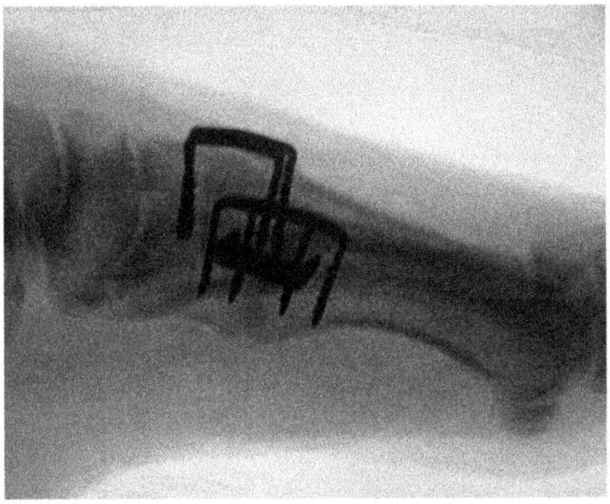

Figure 7. Lateral intra-operative radiograph depicting a 1st/2nd/3rd tarsometatarsal joint fusion with a 90-90-degree configuration technique for the 1st TMTJ.

Furthermore, recent evidence on Lisfranc injuries has demonstrated that the use of CCIs for primary arthrodesis could result in shorter tourniquet times and improved union rates when compared to plate-and-screw constructs [13]. In our series of six patients who underwent fusion for their Lisfranc injuries, we demonstrated promising results with minimal complications. Those findings are in line with the most recent literature [13].

Regarding flat foot deformity correction, based on our experience, we claim that implementing CCI fixation for medialising os calcis osteotomy offers multiple advantages compared to screw fixation. In more detail, for the osteotomy to be meaningful, the appropriate amount of translation has to be maintained, and this can be reliably achieved with CCIs, given the unique design of the calcaneal shift staples.

In terms of talonavicular arthrodesis, a cadaveric study has recently demonstrated that fixation with a combination of 5.5 mm cannulated screw with a nitinol compression staple is advantageous over fixation with a single 5.5 mm screw from a biomechanical point of view [18]. In more detail, higher failure load, stiffness, and cycles to failure were noted in the staple–screw group [19].

3.6. *Relative Contraindications for Nitinol Staples*

Concerning the first metatarsophalangeal joint fusion, in our practice, we tend to avoid CCIs given the fact that the biomechanical and clinical evidence on nitinol staple constructs has not been promising as of yet [11,20].

Furthermore, we advise caution when attempting to span multiple joints with nitinol staples and when it comes to comminuted fractures. Finally, we strongly recommend against orthopaedic surgeons using CCIs for osteoporotic patients, as the compression is questionable in these circumstances, thus increasing the risk of nonunion. Based on six published papers, the rate of complications overall was found to be 11.25% [21]. On the other side, when it comes to poor soft tissue quality, staples are an effective alternative. Likewise, when extensive scarring from previous procedures exists, staples might be a viable option.

3.7. *Removing CCIs*

We wish to draw the readers' attention to the fact that CCIs should not be left proud. Osteophytes and bony prominences are the main culprits in prominent staples, which could then lead to irritation, thus requiring removal. In these circumstances, we highly recommend the careful preparation of the bony bed with rongeurs and/or chisels to achieve an even surface, which will allow for the staples to sit flush with the bone.

From a technical point of view, when planning the removal of CCIs, one should bear in mind that releasing the continuous compression forces prior to metalwork removal results in an uneventful and straightforward surgical procedure. This is because the CCIs continuously attempt to return to their original closed-shape design, thus rendering removal problematic from a biomechanical perspective. Therefore, to achieve an uneventful removal and decrease surgical time, we suggest that surgeons use the large wire-cutting pliers to cut the bridge of the staple after the staple has been slightly lifted off the bone with the use of a small osteotome, thus allowing for the tension to be effectively released. Subsequently, the two remaining staple pieces can be easily extracted with the use of pliers or rongeurs.

3.8. Limitations of the Work

This study has some limitations. First of all, it is based on the experience of two orthopaedic centres only. Second, we have not presented any clinical data to demonstrate the clinical efficacy of the presented techniques in this paper. There is sufficient evidence to support the efficacy of nitinol staples used either alone or in conjunction with other constructs when it comes to fusion for foot and ankle indications. One of the concerns raised earlier on was that the use of nitinol staples results in an unacceptably high hardware failure rate. This was not the case in the most recent studies in the literature [13,21]. Furthermore, we underline that the orthopaedic literature on nitinol staples is only retrospective in nature, and therefore, caution should be exercised. Last but not least, we advise that caution should be exercised before making conclusions on the existing literature regarding nitinol staple fixation. This is because substantial heterogeneity exists in the studies addressing clinical and radiological outcomes.

3.9. Future Research Implications

First of all, we recommend that large-scale randomised trials be conducted to compare the impact of various staple combinations (i.e., different numbers and sizes of staples), especially for the Chopart joints that exhibit lower fusion rates [13,21]. Moreover, more data are needed to provide recommendations on the impact of patient factors, such as bone quality and graft augmentation, in addition to ideal staple characteristics, including arm/bridge length and number of implants per joint.

4. Conclusions

The use of nitinol staples has gained popularity in foot and ankle surgery recently, given the improvements in implant storage and simplicity of use. Overall, we claim that CCI internal fixation is a safe, reproducible, and reliable method when it comes to foot and ankle conditions, but it requires appropriate pre-operative planning, surgical training, and careful implantation. In our series, we demonstrated that primary fusion for Lisfranc injuries yields satisfactory short-term clinical and radiological results. We underline that more prospective papers are required to provide recommendations on ideal fixation characteristics, especially when it comes to hindfoot surgery.

Funding: This research received no external funding.

Conflicts of Interest: The authors declare no conflict of interest.

References

1. Aiyer, A.; Russell, N.A.; Pelletier, M.H.; Myerson, M.; Walsh, W.R. The Impact of Nitinol Staples on the Compressive Forces, Contact Area, and Mechanical Properties in Comparison to a Claw Plate and Crossed Screws for the First Tarsometatarsal Arthrodesis. *Foot Ankle Spec.* **2016**, *9*, 232–240. [CrossRef] [PubMed]
2. Schipper, O.N.; Ellington, J.K. Nitinol Compression Staples in Foot and Ankle Surgery. *Orthop. Clin. N. Am.* **2019**, *50*, 391–399. [CrossRef] [PubMed]
3. Sands, A.; Zderic, I.; Swords, M.; Gehweiler, D.; Ciric, D.; Roth, C.; Nötzli, C.; Gueorguiev, B. First Tarsometatarsal Joint Fusion in Foot—A Biomechanical Human Anatomical Specimen Analysis with Use of Low-Profile Nitinol Staples Acting as Continuous Compression Implants. *Medicina* **2023**, *59*, 1310. [CrossRef] [PubMed]
4. Russell, N.A.; Regazzola, G.; Aiyer, A.; Nomura, T.; Pelletier, M.H.; Myerson, M.; Walsh, W.R. Evaluation of Nitinol Staples for the Lapidus Arthrodesis in a Reproducible Biomechanical Model. *Front. Surg.* **2015**, *2*, 65. [CrossRef]
5. Hoon, Q.J.; Pelletier, M.H.; Christou, C.; Johnson, K.A.; Walsh, W.R. Biomechanical evaluation of shape-memory alloy staples for internal fixation-an in vitro study. *J. Exp. Orthop.* **2016**, *3*, 19. [CrossRef]
6. McKnight, R.R.; Lee, S.K.; Gaston, R.G. Biomechanical Properties of Nitinol Staples: Effects of Troughing, Effective Leg Length, and 2-Staple Constructs. *J. Hand Surg. Am.* **2019**, *44*, 520.e1–520.e9. [CrossRef]
7. Curenton, T.L.; Davis, B.L.; Darnley, J.E.; Weiner, S.D.; Owusu-Danquah, J.S. Assessing the biomechanical properties of nitinol staples in normal, osteopenic and osteoporotic bone models: A finite element analysis. *Injury* **2021**, *52*, 2820–2826. [CrossRef]
8. Horner, K.; Summerhays, B.; Fiala, K.; Schweser, K.M. Radiographic Evaluation of Isolated Continuous Compression Staples for Akin Osteotomy Fixation. *J. Foot Ankle Surg.* **2023**, *62*, 487–491. [CrossRef]
9. Carlsson, Å.S.; Onsten, I.; Besjakov, J.; Sturesson, B. Isolated talo-navicular arthrodesis performed for non-inflammatory conditions blocks motion in healthy adjacent joints—A radiostereometric analysis of 3 cases. *Foot* **1995**, *5*, 80–83. [CrossRef]
10. Carranza-Bencano, A.; Tejero, S.; Fernández Torres, J.J.; Del Castillo-Blanco, G.; Alegrete-Parra, A. Isolated talonavicular joint arthrodesis through minimal incision surgery. *Foot Ankle Surg.* **2015**, *21*, 171–177. [CrossRef]
11. Zhao, J.Z.; Ingall, E.M.; Ritter, Z.; Kwon, J.Y. Radiographically Occult Nonunions After Application of Nitinol Compression Staples: A Report of 3 Cases. *Foot Ankle Int.* **2022**, *43*, 867–871. [CrossRef] [PubMed]
12. Schipper, O.N.; Ford, S.E.; Moody, P.W.; Van Doren, B.; Ellington, J.K. Radiographic Results of Nitinol Compression Staples for Hindfoot and Midfoot Arthrodeses. *Foot Ankle Int.* **2018**, *39*, 172–179. [CrossRef] [PubMed]
13. Dombrowsky, A.R.; Strickland, C.D.; Walsh, D.F.; Hietpas, K.; Conti, M.S.; Irwin, T.A.; Cohen, B.E.; Ellington, J.K.; Jones, C.P., 3rd; Shawen, S.B.; et al. Nitinol Staple Use in Primary Arthrodesis of Lisfranc Fracture-Dislocations. *Foot Ankle Int.* **2024**, *45*, 690–697. [CrossRef]
14. Wang, T.; Pelletier, M.; Johnson, J.; Kline, C.; Walsh, W.; Lareau, C.; Safranski, D. Biomechanical Performance of 4-Leg Sustained Dynamic Compression Staples in First Tarsometatarsal Arthrodesis. *Foot Ankle Spec.* **2024**. *ahead of print*. [CrossRef]
15. Garlapaty, A.; Cook, J.L.; Bezold, W.; Schweser, K. Activated nitinol compression staples are associated with favorable biomechanical properties for talonavicular arthrodesis. *J. Orthop.* **2024**, *52*, 90–93. [CrossRef]
16. Arumugam, V.; Ranjit, S.; Patel, S.; Welck, M. What is the best fixation technique for isolated talonavicular arthrodesis?—A systematic review. *Foot* **2023**, *54*, 101966. [CrossRef]
17. Dock, C.C.; Freeman, K.L.; Coetzee, J.C.; McGaver, R.S.; Giveans, M.R. Outcomes of Nitinol Compression Staples in Tarsometatarsal Fusion. *Foot Ankle Orthop.* **2020**, *5*, 2473011420944904. [CrossRef]
18. O'Neil, J.T.; Abbasi, P.; Parks, B.G.; Miller, S.D. Staple-Plate Plus Screw vs Screw Alone in Talonavicular Arthrodesis: A Cadaveric Biomechanical Study. *Foot Ankle Int.* **2020**, *41*, 1427–1431. [CrossRef]
19. Sleiman, A.; Bejcek, C.; Nestler, A.; Revelt, N.; Thuppal, S.; Mills, A.; Gardner, M. The history of orthopaedic use of nitinol compression staples. *Injury* **2023**, *54*, 111036. [CrossRef]
20. Schafer, K.A.; Baldini, T.; Hamati, M.; Backus, J.D.; Hunt, K.J.; McCormick, J.J. Two Orthogonal Nitinol Staples and Combined Nitinol Staple-Screw Constructs for a First Metatarsophalangeal Joint Arthrodesis: A Biomechanical Cadaver Study. *Foot Ankle Int.* **2022**, *43*, 1493–1500. [CrossRef]
21. Reddy, A.R.; Hampton, H.; Dzieza, W.K.; Toussaint, R.J. Nitinol Compression Staples in Foot Orthopaedic Surgery: A Systematic Review. *Foot Ankle Orthop.* **2024**, *9*, 24730114241300158. [CrossRef] [PubMed]

MDPI AG
Grosspeteranlage 5
4052 Basel
Switzerland
Tel.: +41 61 683 77 34

Journal of Clinical Medicine Editorial Office
E-mail: jcm@mdpi.com
www.mdpi.com/journal/jcm

www.ingramcontent.com/pod-product-compliance
Lightning Source LLC
Chambersburg PA
CBHW062103220926
51850CB00010B/2875
9783725848737